Child Developme
D-score

Children learn to walk, speak, and think at an astonishing pace. The D-score presents a unified framework that places children and their developmental milestones from different tools onto the same scale, enabling comparisons in child development across populations, groups and individuals. This pioneering text explains why we need the D-score, how we construct it, and how we calculate it. It will be of interest not just to professionals in child development, but also to policymakers in international settings and to data scientists.

Stef van Buuren, PhD, is a professor of Statistical Analysis of Incomplete Data at the University of Utrecht and statistician at the Netherlands Organisation for Applied Scientific Research TNO in Leiden. His interests include the analysis of incomplete data and child growth and development (h-index 61). Van Buuren is the inventor of the MICE algorithm for multiple imputation of missing data (>85.000 downloads per month) and has written the accessible monograph *Flexible Imputation of Missing Data*. Second Edition, CRC/Chapman & Hall. He designed the growth charts for the Dutch child health care system and invented the D-score, a new method for expressing child development on a quantitative scale. He consults for the World Health Organization and the Bill & Melinda Gates Foundation. More background at https://stefvanbuuren.name and software at https://github.com/stefvanbuuren.

Iris Eekhout, PhD, holds a double masters in clinical psychology and methodology and statistics of psychology (Leiden University). She obtained her PhD at the Department of Epidemiology and Biostatistics of the VU University medical centre in Amsterdam. Her dissertation work resulted in novel ways of dealing with missing data in questionnaire items and total scores. Currently, Iris teaches a course on missing data analysis in the epidemiology master's program at VU University medical centre. At TNO, Iris works on a variety of projects as a methodologist and statistical analyst related to child health, e. g., measuring child development (D-score) and adaptive screenings for psycho-social problems (psycat). More background at https://www.iriseekhout.com and software at https://github.com/iriseekhout.

Child Development with the D-score

Edited by
Stef van Buuren[1,2] and Iris Eekhout[1]

[1]Netherlands Organisation for Applied Scientific Research TNO, Leiden, 2316 ZL, The Netherlands

[2]University of Utrecht, Utrecht, 3584 CH, The Netherlands

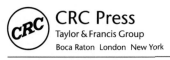

CRC Press
Taylor & Francis Group
Boca Raton London New York

CRC Press is an imprint of the
Taylor & Francis Group, an **informa** business

Designed cover image: shutterstock

First published 2024
by CRC Press
6000 Broken Sound Parkway NW, Suite 300, Boca Raton, FL 33487-2742

and by CRC Press
4 Park Square, Milton Park, Abingdon, Oxon, OX14 4RN

CRC Press is an imprint of Taylor & Francis Group, LLC

Library of Congress Cataloging-in-Publication Data
A catalog record has been requested for this book

ISBN: 978-1-003-21631-5 (ebk)
ISBN: 978-1-032-10634-2 (hbk)
ISBN: 978-1-032-10633-5 (pbk)

DOI: 10.1201/9781003216315

Typeset in Times New Roman
by T&F Books

Contents

1 Child development with the D-score: turning milestones into measurement

2   Child development with the D-score: tuning instruments to unity

Illustrations

TABLES

Contributors

Maureen Black University of Maryland School of Medicine, Baltimore, MD, USA

Marianne de Wolff Netherlands Organisation for Applied Scientific Research TNO, Leiden, The Netherlands

Manon Grevinga Netherlands Organisation for Applied Scientific Research TNO, Leiden, The Netherlands

Maria C. Olthof University of Amsterdam, The Netherlands

Paula van Dommelen Netherlands Organisation for Applied Scientific Research TNO, Leiden, The Netherlands

Preface

Maureen M. Black[1,2]
[1]Department of Pediatrics and Department of Epidemiology and Public Health, University of Maryland School of Medicine, Maryland, USA
[2]RTI International, North Carolina, USA

ABSTRACT

The foundations of adult health and wellbeing have their origins early in life, often measured by children's early growth and development. A valid and easily interpretable metric is needed to interpret the underlying latent construct of early childhood development that can represent change and is comparable across cultures and contexts.

KEYWORDS: CHILD DEVELOPMENT; D-SCORE

The foundations of adult health and wellbeing have their origins early in life, often measured by children's early growth and development (Clark *et al.*, 2020). Growth standards established by the World Health Organization (WHO) have been adopted globally and are used as indices and targets for improvement. For example, in 2018, 219 million children under 5 years of age (21.9%) were stunted (height for age < -2 standard deviations of the WHO growth standards) (UNICEF, 2019). Stunting early in life has been associated with negative childhood development, academic achievement, and adult productivity. In the absence of direct population-based metrics for childhood development, stunting and poverty have been used as proxy indicators to estimate the number of children not reaching their developmental potential (Lu *et al.*, 2016).

Although stunting and poverty have been effective indicators and have contributed to advances in global childhood development policies and programs (Black *et al.*, 2017), they lack the sensitivity to measure changes associated with programmatic interventions. Early childhood development is a latent construct composed of an ordinal sequence of developmental domains (motor, language, cognitive, personal-social). A valid and easily interpretable metric is needed to interpret the underlying latent construct of early childhood development that can represent change and is comparable across cultures and contexts. Chapter 1 - Turning milestones into measurement - shows that the D-score (Developmental score) meets those criteria.

Chapter 2 - Tuning instruments to unity - deals with the problem of how to define and calculate the D-score from data obtained from multiple studies and multiple instruments. After harmonizing longitudinal measures of childhood

DOI: 10.12688/gatesopenres.13316.1

development among over 36,000 children from 11 countries (Weber *et al.*, 2019), the statistical analysis produced a D-score scale with interval qualities that can reflect change over time and enable within and across country comparisons. In addition, the D-score is responsive to environmental conditions that may impact children's development, ranging from community programs and policies to macro-level conditions from migration, inequities, or climate. Applied to populations, direct metrics of children's early growth and development assess the current status of the population's health and well-being, establish predictions of future health and well-being, and provide opportunities to measure changes. Thus, applying the D-score to the early development of children extends to populations and society as a whole.

Maureen M. Black (July, 2020)

REFERENCES

Black MM, Walker SP, Fernald LCH, *et al.*: Early Childhood Development Coming of Age: Science Through the Life Course. *Lancet.* 2017; 389(10064): 77–90. 2771761410.1016/S0140-6736(16)31389-75884058

Clark H, Coll-Seck AM, Banerjee A, *et al.*: A Future for the World's Children? A WHO–UNICEF–Lancet Commission. *Lancet.* 2020; 395(10224): 605–658. 3208582110.1016/S0140-6736(19)32540-1

Lu C, Black MM, Richter LM: Risk of Poor Development in Young Children in Low-Income and Middle-Income Countries: An Estimation and Analysis at the Global, Regional, and Country Level. *Lancet Glob Health.* 2016; 4(12): e916–22. 2771763210.1016/S2214-109X(16)30266-25881401

UNICEF: The State of the World's Children 2019: Children, Food and Nutrition: Growing Well in a Changing World. *UNICEF.* 2019.Reference Source

Weber AM, Rubio-Codina M, Walker SP, *et al.*: The D-score: A Metric for Interpreting the Early Development of Infants and Toddlers Across Global Settings. *BMJ Glob Health.* 2019; 4(6): e001724. 3180350810.1136/bmjgh-2019-0017246882553

1

Child development with the D-score: turning milestones into measurement

Edited by
Stef van Buuren[1,2] and Iris Eekhout[1]
[1]Netherlands Organisation for Applied Scientific Research TNO, Leiden, 2316 ZL, The Netherlands
[2]University of Utrecht, Utrecht, 3584 CH, The Netherlands

1.1 Introduction

Stef van Buuren[1,2]
Iris Eekhout[1]
with Marianne de Wolff
[1]Netherlands Organisation for Applied Scientific
Research TNO, Leiden, 2316 ZL, The Netherlands
[2]University of Utrecht, Utrecht, 3584 CH, The
Netherlands

This introductory section outlines why we utilize the D-score:

- reviewing key discussions about the first 1000 days in a child's life (1.1.1)
- highlighting the relevance of early childhood development for later life (1.1.2)
- discussing the use of stunting as a proxy for development (1.1.3)
- pointing to existing instruments to quantify neurocognitive development (1.1.4)
- explaining why we have written this chapter (1.1.5)
- delineating the intended audience (1.1.6)

1.1.1 FIRST 1000 DAYS

The *first 1000 days* refers to the time needed for a child to grow from conception to the second birthday. It is a time of rapid change. During this period the architecture of the developing brain is very open to the influence of relationships and experiences (Shonkhoff *et al.*, 2016). Early experiences affect the nature and quality of the brain's developing architecture by reinforcing some synapses and pruning others through lack of use. The first 1000 days shape the brain's architecture, but higher-order brain functions continue to develop into adolescence and early adulthood (Kolb *et al.*, 2017).

The classic *nature versus nurture debate* contrasts the viewpoints that variation in development is primarily due to either genetic or environmental differences. The current scientific consensus is that both genetic predisposition and ecological differences influence all traits (Rutter, 2007). The environment in which a child develops (before and soon after birth) provides experiences that can modify gene activity (Caspi *et al.*, 2010). Negative influences, such as exposure to stressful life circumstances or environmental toxins may leave a *chemical signature* on the genes, thereby influencing how genes work in that individual.

During the first 1000 days, infants are highly dependent on their caregivers to protect them from adversities and to help them regulate their physiology and

DOI: 10.1201/9781003216315-1

behavior. As Figure 1.1.1 illustrates, caregivers can do this through responsive care, including routines for sleeping and feeding. To reach their developmental potential, children require nutrition, responsive caregiving, opportunities to explore and learn, and protection from environmental threats (Black *et al.*, 2017). Gradually, children build self-regulatory skills that enable them to manage stress as they interact with the world around them (Johnson *et al.*, 2013).

1.1.2   RELEVANCE OF CHILD DEVELOPMENT

The first 1000 days is a time of rapid change. Early experiences affect brain development and influence lifelong learning and health (Shonkhoff *et al.*, 2016). Healthy development is associated with future school achievement, well-being, and success in life (Bellman *et al.*, 2013).

Professionals and parents consider it important to monitor children's development. Tracking child development enables professionals to identify children with signs of potential delay. Timely identification can help children and their parents to benefit from early intervention. In a normal population, developmental delay affects about 1–3% of children. A delay in development may indicate underlying disorders. About 1% of children have an autism spectrum disorder (Baird *et al.*, 2006), 1–2% a mild learning disability, and 5–10% have a specific learning disability in a single domain (Horridge, 2011).

Children develop at different rates, and it is vital to distinguish those who are within the "normal" range from those who are following a more pathological

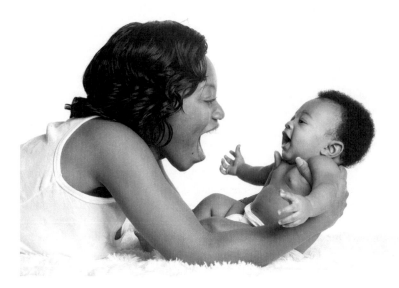

FIGURE 1.1.1   Serve and return interactions shape brain architecture.

Source: Shutterstock, under license.

course (Bellman *et al.*, 2013). There is good evidence that early identification and early intervention improve the outcomes of children (Britto *et al.*, 2017). Early intervention is crucial for children with developmental disabilities because barriers to healthy development early in life impede progress at each subsequent stage.

Monitoring child development provides caregivers and parents with reliable information about the child and an opportunity to intervene at an early age. Understanding the developmental health of populations of children allows organizations and policymakers to make informed decisions about programmes that support children's greatest needs (Bellman *et al.*, 2013).

1.1.3   STUNTING AS PROXY FOR CHILD DEVELOPMENT

Stunting is the impaired physical growth and development that children experience from poor nutrition, repeated infection, and inadequate psychosocial stimulation. Linear growth in children is commonly expressed as length-for-age or height-for-age in comparison to normative growth standards (Wit *et al.*, 2017). According to the World Health Organization (WHO), children are stunted if their height-for-age is more than two standard deviations below the Child Growth Standards median. Stunting caused by chronic nutritional deprivation in early childhood is as an indicator of child development (Perkins *et al.*, 2017).

There is consistent evidence for an association between stunting and poor child development, despite heterogeneity in the estimation of its magnitude (Miller *et al.*, 2016; Sudfeld *et al.*, 2015). Considering impaired linear growth as a proxy measure for child development is easy to do, and quite common. Yet, using impaired height growth as a measure for child development is not without limitations:

- The relation between height and child development is weak after adjustment for age;
- Height is a physical indicator that does not take into account a direct evaluation of a child's cognitive or mental performance;
- There is considerable heterogeneity in heights of children all over the world;
- Height is not sensitive to rapid changes in child development.

1.1.4   MEASURING NEUROCOGNITIVE DEVELOPMENT

Assessment of early neurocognitive development in children is challenging for many reasons (Ellingsen, 2016). During the first years of life, developmental change occurs rapidly, and the manifestation of different skills and abilities varies considerably across children. Moreover, a child's performance on a cognitive task is very susceptible to measurement setting, timing and the health of the child that day.

Recently, a toolkit was published that reviews 147 assessment tools developed for children ages 0–8 years in low- and middle-income countries (Fernald *et al.*, 2017). Some of the most widely used tools include the Ages & Stages Questionnaires (ASQ), Achenbach Child Behavior Checklist (CBCL), Bayley Scales of Infant Development (BSID), Denver Developmental Screening Test (DEN), Griffiths Scales of Child Development (GRF), Mullen Scale of Early Learning (MSEL), Strengths and Difficulties Questionnaire (SDQ), Wechsler Intelligence Scale for Children (WISC), and its younger age counterpart Wechsler Preschool and Primary Scale of Intelligence (WPPSI).

Each of these tools has its strengths and limitations. For example, the ASQ and DEN are screeners for general child development. The CBCL and SDQ are screeners for behavioral and mental health, not cognition or general development. DEN is relatively easy and quick to administer, but not very precise. It is out of production, not being sold or re-normed. The BSID, MSEL, and GRF provide a clinical assessment at the individual level and requires a skilled professional to administer. Some instruments collect observations through the caregiver (ASQ), whereas others emphasize traits and behavior over performance (SDQ, CBCL). Also, the age ranges to which the instruments are sensitive vary. Furthermore, they may cover different domains of development.

The ideal child development assessment would be easy to administer and has high reliability, validity, and cross-cultural appropriateness. It should also show appropriate sensitivity in scores at different ages and ability levels. It is no surprise that no test can meet all of these criteria. Many tests are too long, difficult to administer, lack cross-cultural validity, or have low reliability. Also, many instruments are proprietary and costly to use.

1.1.5   WHY THIS CHAPTER?

We believe that **there cannot be one instrument** for measuring child development that is suitable for all situations. In general, the tool needs tailoring to the setting. For example, to find a delayed child, we need an instrument that is precise for that individual child, and that is sensitive to different domains of delay. In contrast, if we want to estimate the proportion of children that is *developmentally on track* in a region, we need one culturally unbiased, relatively imprecise low-cost measurement made on many children across many ages. The optimal instrument will look quite different in both cases.

We also believe that **there can be one scale** for measuring child development and that this scale is useful for many applications. Such a scale is similar to well-known measures for body height, body weight or body temperature. These measurements have a clearly defined unit (i.e., centimetre, kilogram, degree Celsius), which moreover is assumed to be constant across all scale locations. We express measurements as the number of scale units (e.g. 92 cm). Note that there may be multiple instruments for measuring a child height (e.g. ruler, laser distance meter, echolocation, ability to reach the door handle, and so on). Still, their result translates into scale units (cm here). The opposite is also true, and perhaps more familiar. We may have one instrument and express the result in multiple units (e.g. cm, inches, light-years).

Instruments and scales are different things. Currently, instruments for measuring child development define their own scales, which renders the measurements made by distinct tools incomparable. No measurement unit for child development yet exists. It would undoubtedly be an advance if we could tailor the measurement instrument to the setting while retaining the advantage of a scale with a clearly defined unit across different tools. We can then compare the data collected by distinct devices. This chapter explores the theory and practice for making that happen.

1.1.6   INTENDED AUDIENCE

We aim for three broad audiences:

- Professionals in the field of child growth and development;
- Policymakers in international settings;
- Statisticians, methodologists, and data scientists.

Professionals in child development will become familiar with a new approach to measuring child development in early childhood. We plan to separate the measurement instrument from the scale used to express the result. This formulation allows the user **to select the instrument most suited for a particular setting**. Since instruments differ widely in age coverage, length, administration mode, and domain coverage (Boggs *et al.*, 2019), the ability to choose the instrument, while not giving up comparability, represents a significant advance over routines that marry the scale to the instrument.

Policymakers in international settings wish to know the effect of different interventions on child development. Gaining insight into such effects is not so easy since different studies use different instruments. The ability to place measurements made by different instruments onto the same scale will allow for a **more accurate understanding of policy effects**. It also enables the setting of priorities and actions that are less dependent on the way the data were collected.

Statisticians and data scientists generally prefer numeric values with an unambiguous unit (e.g., centimeters, kilograms) over a vector of dichotomous data points. This chapter shows how to convert a series of PASS/FAIL scores to a numeric value with interval scale properties. The existence of such a scale opens the way for the **application of precise analytic techniques**, similar to those applied to child height and body weight. The techniques have a solid psychometric backing, and also apply to other types of problems.

1.2 Short history

Stef van Buuren[1,2]
Iris Eekhout[1]
[1]Netherlands Organisation for Applied Scientific
Research TNO, Leiden, 2316 ZL, The Netherlands
[2]University of Utrecht, Utrecht, 3584 CH, The
Netherlands

The measurement of child development has quite an extensive history. This section

- reviews definitions of child development (1.2.1)
- discusses concepts in the nature of child development (1.2.2)
- shows a classic example of motor measurements (1.2.3)
- summarizes typical questions whose answers need proper measurements (1.2.4)

1.2.1 WHAT IS CHILD DEVELOPMENT?

In contrast to concepts like height or temperature, it is unclear what exactly constitutes child development. Shirley (1931) executed one of the first rigorous studies in the field with the explicit aim

> that the many aspects of development, anatomical, physical, motor, intellectual, and emotional, be studied simultaneously.

Shirley gave empirical definitions of each of these domains of development.

Certain domains advance through a fixed sequence. Figure 1.2.1 illustrates the various stages needed for going from a *fetal posture* to *walking alone*. The ages are indicative of when these events happen, but there is a considerable variation in timing between infants.

Gesell (1943) (p. 88) formulated the following definition of development:

> Development is a continuous process that proceeds stage by stage in an orderly sequence.

Gesell's definition emphasizes that development is a continuous process. The stages are useful as indicators to infer the level of maturity but are of limited interest by themselves.

Liebert *et al.* (1974) (p. 5) emphasized that development is not a phenomenon that unfolds in isolation.

DOI: 10.1201/9781003216315-2

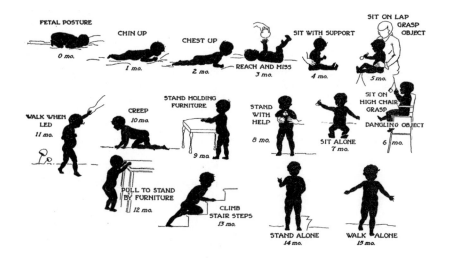

FIGURE 1.2.1   Gross motor development as a sequence of milestones.
Source: Shirley (1933), with permission.

Development refers to a process in growth and capability over time, as a function of both maturation and interaction with the environment.

Cameron & Bogin (2012) (p. 11) defined an endpoint of development, as follows:

"Growth" is defined as an increase in size, while "maturity" or "development" is an increase in functional ability...The endpoint of maturity is when a human is functionally able to procreate successfully ... not just biological maturity but also behavioural and perhaps social maturity.

Berk (2011) (p. 30) presented a dynamic systems perspective on child development as follows:

Development cannot be characterized as a single line of change, and is more like a web of fibres branching out in many directions, each representing a different skill area that may undergo both continuous and stagewise transformation.

There are many more definitions of child development. The ones described here illustrate the main points of view in the field.

1.2.2   THEORIES OF CHILD DEVELOPMENT

The field of child development is vast and spans multiple academic disciplines. This short overview, therefore, cannot do justice to the enormous richness.

Readers new to the field might orient themselves by browsing through an introductory academic titles (Berk, 2011; Santrock, 2011), or by searching for the topic of interest in an encyclopedia, e.g., Salkind (2002).

The introductions by Santrock (2011) and Berk (2011) both distinguish major theories in child development according to how each answer to following three questions:

1.2.2.1 CONTINUOUS OR DISCONTINUOUS?

Does development evolve gradually as a continuous process or are there qualitatively distinct stages, with jumps occurring from one step to another?

Many stage-based theories of human development have been proposed over the years: social and emotional development by psycho-sexual stages introduced by Freud and furthered by Erikson (Erikson, 1963), Kohlberg's six stages of moral development (Kohlberg, 1984) and Piaget's cognitive development theory (Piaget & Inhelder, 1969). Piaget distinguishes four main periods throughout childhood. The first period, the *sensorimotor period* (approximately 0–2 years), is subdivided into six stages. When taken together, these six stages describe "the road to conceptual thought." Piaget's stages are qualitatively different and aim to unravel the mechanism involved in intellectual development.

On the other hand, Gesell and others emphasize development as a continuous process. Gesell (1943) (p. 88) says:

> A stage represents a degree or level of maturity in the cycle of development. A
> stage is simply a passing moment, while development, like time, keeps marching on.

1.2.2.2 ONE COURSE OR MULTIPLE PARALLEL TRACKS?

Stage theorists assume that children progress sequentially through the same set of stages. This assumption is also explicit in the work of Gesell.

The ecological and dynamic systems theories view development as continuous, though not necessarily progressing in an orderly fashion, so there may be multiple, parallel ways to reach the same point. The developmental path taken by a given child will depend on the child's unique combination of personal and environmental circumstances, including cultural diversity in development.

1.2.2.3 NATURE OR NURTURE?

Figure 1.2.2 illustrates that children vary in appearance. Are genetic or environmental factors more important for influencing development? Most theories generally acknowledge the role of both but differ in emphasis. In practice, the debate centres on the question of how to explain individual differences.

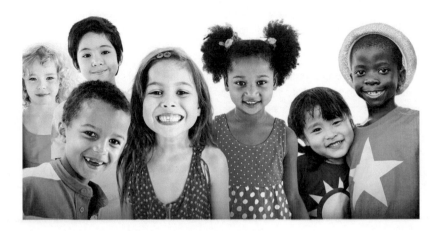

FIGURE 1.2.2 A group of culturally diverse children.

Source: Shutterstock, under license.

Maturation is the process of becoming fully developed, much like the natural unfolding of a flower. The process depends on both genetic factors (species, breed) as well as environmental influences (sunlight, water, nutrition). Some theorists emphasize that differences in child development are innate and stable over time, although there may be differences in unfolding speed due to different environments. Others argue that environmental factors drive differences in development between children, and changing these factors could very well impact child development.

Our position in this debate has practical implications. If we believe that differences are natural and stable, then it may not make much sense trying to change the environment, as the impact on development is likely to be small. On the other hand, we may consider developmental potential as evenly distributed, with its expression governed by the environment. In the latter case, improving life circumstances may have substantial pay-offs in terms of better development.

1.2.3 EXAMPLE OF MOTOR DEVELOPMENT

1.2.3.1 SHIRLEY'S MOTOR DATA

For illustration, we use data on locomotor development from a classic study on child development among 25 babies. Shirley (1931) collected measurements of the baby's walking ability, starting at ages around 13 weeks, in an ingenious way. The investigator lays out a white paper of twelve inches wide on the floor of the living room, and lightly greases the soles of the baby's feet with olive oil.

The baby was invited to "walk" on the sheet. Of course, very young infants need substantial assistance. Footprints left were later coloured by graphite and measured. Measurements during the first year were repeated every week or bi-weekly.

Table 1.2.1 (Shirley, 1931, Appendix 8) lists the age (in weeks) of the 21 babies when they started, respectively, stepping, standing, walking with help, and walking alone. Blanks indicate missing data. A blank in the first column means that the baby was already stepping when the observation started (Virginia Ruth, Sibyl, Donovan, Torey and Doris). Max and Martin, who have blanks in the second column, skipped standing and went directly from stepping to walking with help. Doris has a blank in the last column because she passed away before she could walk alone.

1.2.3.2 INDIVIDUAL TRAJECTORIES OF MOTOR DEVELOPMENT

Figure 1.2.3 is a visual representation of the information in Table 1.2.1. Each data point is the age of the first occurrence of the next stage. Before that age, we assume the baby is in the previous stage.

TABLE 1.2.1
Age at beginning stages of walking (in weeks) for 21 babies.

Name	Sex	Stepping	Standing	Walking with help	Walking alone
Martin	boy	15		21	50
Carol	girl	15	19	37	50
Max	boy	14		25	54
Virginia Ruth	girl		21	41	54
Sibyl	girl		22	37	58
David	boy	19	27	34	60
James D.	boy	19	30	45	60
Harvey	boy	14	27	42	62
Winnifred	girl	15	30	41	62
Quentin	boy	15	23	38	64
Maurice	boy	18	23	45	66
Judy	girl	18	29	45	66
Irene May	girl	19	34	45	66
Peter	boy	15	29	49	66
Walley	boy	18	33	54	68
Fred	boy	15	32	46	70
Donovan	boy		23	50	70
Patricia	girl	15	30	45	70
Torey	boy		21	72	74
Larry	boy	13	41	54	76
Doris	girl		23	44	

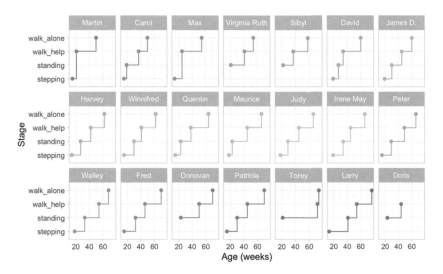

FIGURE 1.2.3 Staircase plot indicating the age at which each baby achieves a new milestone of gross-motor functioning.

Figure 1.2.3 makes it easy to spot the quick walkers (Martin, Carol) and slow walkers (Patricia, Torey, Larry). Furthermore, we may also locate children who remain a long time in a particular stage (Torey, Larry) or who jump over stages (Martin, Max).

For ease of plotting, the categories on the vertical axis are equally spaced. The height of the jump from one stage to the next has no sensible interpretation. We might be inclined to think that the vertical distance portrays to how difficult it is to achieve the next stage, but this is inaccurate. Instead, the ability needed to set the next step corresponds to the *horizontal line length* between stages. For example, on average, the line for stepping is rather short in all plots, so going from stepping to standing is relatively easy.

Figure 1.2.3 presents data from only those visits where a jump occurred. The number of house visits made during the ages of 0–2 years was far higher. Shirley (1931) collected data from 1370 visits, whereas Figure 1.2.3 plot only the 76 occasions that showed a jump. Thus the data collection needs to be intense and costly to obtain individual curves. Fortunately, there are alternatives that are much more efficient.

1.2.4 TYPICAL QUESTIONS ASKED IN CHILD DEVELOPMENT

The emotional, social and physical development of the young child has a direct effect on the adult he or she will become. We may be interested in measuring child development for answering clinical, policy or public health questions.

Table 1.2.2 lists typical questions whose answers require measuring child development. Note that all questions compare the amount of child development between groups or time points. A few questions compare development for the same child, group or population at different ages. Others compare development at the same age across different children, groups or populations.

TABLE 1.2.2

Questions whose answers require quantitative measurements of child development.

Level	Question
Individual	What is the child's gain in development since the last visit?
Individual	What is the difference in development between the child and peers of the same age?
Individual	How does the child's development compare to a norm?
Group	What is the effect of this intervention on child development?
Group	What is the difference in child development between these two groups?
Population	What is the change in average child development since the last measurement?
Population	What was the effect of implementing this policy on child development?
Population	How does this country compare to other countries in terms of child development?

1.3 Quantifying child development

Stef van Buuren[1,2]
Iris Eekhout[1]
[1]Netherlands Organisation for Applied Scientific Research TNO, Leiden, 2316 ZL, The Netherlands
[2]University of Utrecht, Utrecht, 3584 CH, The Netherlands

This section discusses four principles to quantify child development:

- Age-based measurement (1.3.1)
- Probability-based measurement (1.3.2)
- Score-based measurement (1.3.3)
- Unit-based measurement (1.3.4)

1.3.1 AGE-BASED MEASUREMENT OF DEVELOPMENT

1.3.1.1 MOTIVATION FOR AGE-BASED MEASUREMENT

Milestones form the based building blocks for instruments to measure child development. Methods to quantify growth using separate milestones relate the milestone behaviour to the child's age. Gesell (1943) (p. 89) formulated this goal as follows:

> We think of behaviour in terms of age, and we think of age in terms of behaviour. For any selected age it is possible to sketch a portrait which delineates the behaviour characteristics typical of the age.

There is an extensive literature that quantifies development in terms of the ages at which the child is expected to show a specific behaviour. The oldest methods for quantifying child development calculate an *age equivalent* for achieving a milestone, and compare the child's age to this age equivalent.

1.3.1.2 AGE EQUIVALENT AND DEVELOPMENTAL AGE

Figure 1.3.1 graphs the ages at which each of the 21 children enter a given stage in Shirley's motor data of Table 1.2.1. Since `standing` follows `stepping`, children who can stand are older than the children who are stepping. Hence the ages for standing are located more to the right.

DOI: 10.1201/9781003216315-3

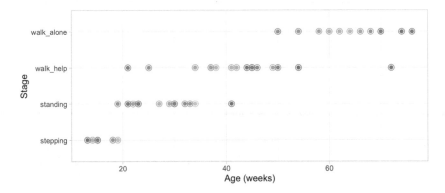

FIGURE 1.3.1   Ages at which 21 children achieve four motor development milestones.

Since age and development are so intimately related, we can express the *difficulty* of a milestone as the *mean age* at which children achieve it. For example, Stott (1967) (p. 25) defines the *age equivalent* and its use for measurement, as follows:

> The age equivalent of a particular stage is simply the average age at which children reach that particular stage.

Figure 1.3.2 adds the mean age and the boxplot at which the children enter the four stages. The difficulty of these milestones can thus be expressed as age equivalents: 16.1 weeks for stepping, 27.2 weeks for standing, 43.3 weeks for walking with help and 63.3 weeks for walking alone.

Thus, a child that is stepping beyond the age of 16.1 weeks is considered later than average, whereas a child already stepping before 27.2 weeks earlier than average. We may also calculate age delta as the difference between the child's age and the norm age, and express it as "two weeks late" or "three

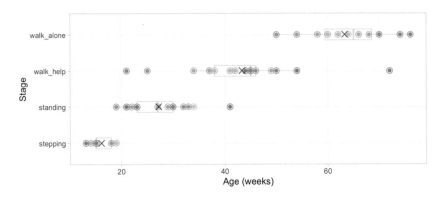

FIGURE 1.3.2   Mean (symbol x) and spread of the ages at which 21 children achieve four motor development milestones.

weeks ahead." Summarizing age delta's over different milestones has led to concepts like *developmental age* as a measure of a child's development.

1.3.1.3 LIMITATIONS OF AGE-BASED MEASUREMENT

Age-based measurement is easy to understand, and widely used in the popular press, but not without pitfalls:

1. Age-based measurement requires us to know the ages at which the child entered a new stage. The mean age can be a biased estimate of item difficulty if visits are widely apart, irregular or missing.
2. Age-based measurement can inform us whether a child is achieving a given milestone early of late. However, it does not tell us what behaviours are characteristic for children of a given age.
3. Age-based measurement cannot exist without an age norm. When there are no norms, we cannot quantify development.
4. Age-based measurement works only at the item level. Although we may average age delta's over milestones, the choice of milestones is arbitrary.

1.3.2 PROBABILITY-BASED MEASUREMENT

An alternative is to calculate the *probability* of achieving a milestone at a given age and compare the child's response to that probability.

The passing probability is an interpretable and relevant measure. An operational advantage of the approach is that the necessary calculations place fewer demands on the available data and can be done even for cross-sectional studies.

1.3.2.1 EXAMPLE OF PROBABILITY-BASED MEASUREMENT

Figure 1.3.3 plots the percentage of children achieving each of Shirley's motor stages against age. There are four cumulative curves, one for each milestone, that indicate the percentage of children that pass.

In analogy to the age equivalent introduced in Section 1.3.1.2 we can define the *difficulty* of the milestone as the age at which 50 per cent of the children pass. In the Figure we see that the levels of difficulty are approximately 14.2 weeks (stepping), 27.0 weeks (standing), 43.8 weeks (walking with help) and 64.0 weeks (walking alone). Also, we may easily find the ages at which 10 per cent or 90 per cent of the children pass each milestone.

Observe there is a gradual decline in the steepness as we move from stepping to walk_alone. For example, we need an age interval of 13 weeks (33 - 20) to go from 10 to 90 per cent in standing, but need 19 weeks (71 - 52) to go from 10 to 90 per cent in walking alone. Thus, one step on the age axis corresponds to different increments in probability. The flattening

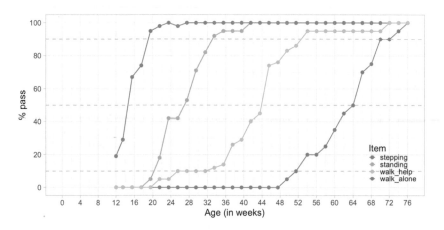

FIGURE 1.3.3   Probability of achieving four motor milestones against age.

pattern is typical for child development and represents evidence that evolution is faster at earlier ages.

1.3.2.2   Limitations of probability-based measurement

Probability-based measurement is a popular way to create instruments for screening on developmental delay. For example, each milestone in the Denver II (Frankenburg *et al.*, 1992) has markers for the 25th, 50th, 75th and 90th age percentile.

1. The same age step corresponds to different probabilities.
2. The measurement cannot exist without some norm population. When norms differ, we cannot compare the measurements.
3. Interpretation is at the milestone level, sometimes supplemented by procedures for counting the number of delays. No aggregate takes all responses into account.

1.3.3   SCORE-BASED MEASUREMENT OF DEVELOPMENT

1.3.3.1   Motivation for score-based measurement

Score-based measurement takes the responses on multiple milestones and counts the total number of items passed as a measure of development. This approach takes all answers into account, hence leading to a more stable result.

One may order milestones in difficulty, and skip those that are too easy, and stop administration for those that are too difficult. In such cases, we cannot merely interpret the sum score of a measure of development. Instead, we need to correct for the subset of administered milestones. The usual working assumption is that the child would have passed all easier milestones and failed on all more difficult ones. We may repeat this procedure for different domains, e.g. motor, cognitive, and so on.

1.3.3.2   EXAMPLE OF SCORE-BASED MEASUREMENT

Figure 1.3.4 is a gross-motor score calculated as the number of milestones passed. It varies from 0 to 3.

The plot suggests that the difference in development between scores 0 and 1 is the same as the difference between, say, scores 2 and 3. *This is not correct.* For example, suppose that we express the difficulty of the milestone as an age-equivalent. From Section 1.3.1.2 we see that the difference between stepping and standing is 27.2 - 16.1 = 11.1 weeks, whereas the difference between walking alone and walking with help is 63.3 - 43.3 = 20 weeks. Thus, according to age equivalents scores 0 and 1 should be closer to each other, and ratings 2 and 3 should be drawn more apart.

1.3.3.3   LIMITATIONS OF SCORE-BASED MEASUREMENT

Score-based measurement is today's dominant approach, but is not without conceptual and logistical issues.

1. The total score depends not only on the actual developmental status of the child, but also on the set of milestones administered. If a milestone is skipped or added, the sum score cannot be interpreted anymore as a measure of developmental status. It might be possible to correct for

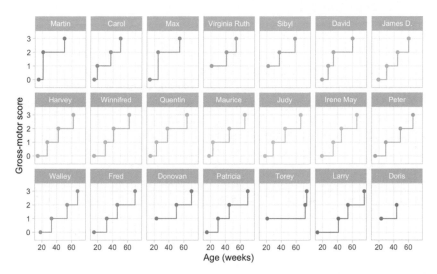

FIGURE 1.3.4 Same data as in Figure 1.2.3, but now with the vertical axis representing gross-motor score.

starting and stopping rules under the assumptions described in Section 1.3.3.1, but such will be involved if intermediate milestones are missing.
2. It is not possible to compare the scores made by different instruments. Some instruments allow conversion to age-conditional scores. However, the sample used to derive such transformations pertain to that tool and does not generalize to others.
3. Domains are hard to separate. For example, some cognitive milestones tap into fine motor capabilities, and vice versa. There are different ways to define domains, so domain interpretation varies by instrument.
4. Administration of a full test may take substantial time. The materials are often proprietary and costly.

1.3.4   UNIT-BASED MEASUREMENT OF DEVELOPMENT

1.3.4.1   MOTIVATION FOR UNIT-BASED MEASUREMENT

Unit-based measurement starts by defining ideal properties and derives a procedure to aggregate the responses on milestones into an overall score that will meet this ideal.

Section 1.2.4 highlighted questions for individuals, groups and populations. There are three questions:

- What is the difference in development over time for the same child, group or community?
- What is the difference in development between different children, groups or populations of the same age?
- How does child development compare to a norm?

In the ideal situation, we would like to have a continuous (latent) variable D (for development) that measures child development. The scale should allow us to quantify *ability* of persons, groups or populations from low to high. It should have a *constant unit* so that a given difference in ability refers to the same quantity across the entire scale. We find the same property in height, where a distance of 10 cm represents the same amount for molecules, people or galaxies. When are these conditions are met, we say that we measure on an *interval scale*.

If we succeed in creating an interval scale for child development, an enormous arsenal of techniques developed for quantitative variables opens up to measure, track and analyze child development. We may then evaluate the status of a child in terms of D points gained, create age-dependent diagrams (just like growth charts for height and weight), devise age-conditional measures for child development, and intelligent adaptive testing schemes. Promising studies on Dutch data (Jacobusse *et al.*, 2006; van Buuren, 2014) suggest that such benefits are well within reach.

1.3.4.2 EXAMPLE OF UNIT-BASED MEASUREMENT

Figure 1.3.5 is similar to Figure 1.3.3, but with `Age` replaced by `Ability`. Also, modelled curves have replaced empirical ones, but this is not essential.

We estimated the ability values on the horizontal axis from the data. The values correspond to the amount of development of each visit. Likewise, we calculated the logistic curves from the data. These reflect the probability of passing each milestone *at a given level of ability.*

Figure 1.3.5 shows that the probability of passing a milestone increases with ability. Items are sorted according to difficulty from left to right. Milestone `stepping` is the easiest and `walk_alone` is the most difficult. The point at which a logistic curve crosses the 50 per cent line (marked by a cross) is the *difficulty of the milestone.*

The increase in ability that is needed to go from 10 to 90 per cent is about five units here. Since all curves are parallel, the interval is constant for all scale locations. Thus, the scale is an *interval scale* with a *constant unit of measurement*, the type of measurement needed for answering the basic questions identified in Section 1.3.4.1.

1.3.4.3 LIMITATIONS OF UNIT-BASED MEASUREMENT

While unit-based measurement has many advantages, it cannot perform miracles.

1. An important assumption is that the milestones "measure the same thing," or put differently, are manifestations of a continuous latent variable that can be measured by empirical observations. Unit-based measurement won't work if there is no sensible latent scale.

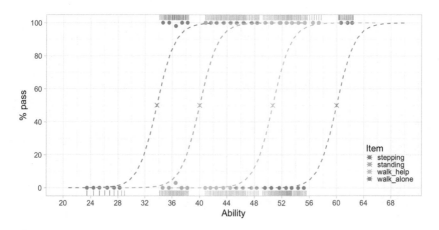

FIGURE 1.3.5 Modelled probability of achieving four motor milestones against the D-score.

2. The portrayed advantages hold only if the discrepancies between the data and the model are relatively small. Since the simplest and most powerful measurement models are strict, it is essential to obtain a good fit between the data and the model.
3. The construction of unit-based measurement requires psychometric expertise, specialized computer software and considerable sample sizes.

1.3.5   A UNIFIED FRAMEWORK

This section brings together the four approaches outlined in this section into a unified framework.

Figure 1.3.6 shows the imaginary positions on a gross-motor continuum of three babies from Figure 1.2.1 at the age of 30 weeks. Both milestones and children are ordered along the same continuum. Thus, standing is more difficult than stepping, and at week 30, Doris is ahead of Walley in terms of motor development.

More generally, measurement is the process of locating milestones and children on a line. This line represents a *latent variable*, a continuous construct that defines the different poles of the concept that we want to measure. A latent variable ranges from low to high.

The first part of measurement is to determine the location of the milestones on the latent variable. In many cases, the instrument maker has already done that. For example, each length marker on a ruler corresponds to a milestone for measuring length. The manufacturer of the ruler has already placed the marks at the appropriate places on the tool, and we take for granted that each marker has been calibrated correctly.

A milestone for child development is similar to a length marker, but

- we may not know how much development the milestone measures, so its location on the line is unknown, or uncertain;
- we may not know whether the milestone measures child development at all so that it may have no location on the line.

The second part of measurement is to find the location of each child on the line. For child height, this is easy: We place the horizontal headpiece on top of the child's head and read off the closest height marker. Since we lack a physical

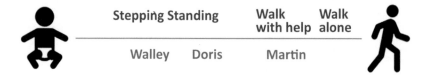

FIGURE 1.3.6   Placing milestones and children onto the same line reveals their positions.

ruler for development, we must deduce the child's location on the line from the responses on a series of well-chosen milestones.

By definition, we cannot observe the values of a latent variable directly. However, we may be able to measure variables (milestones) that are related to the latent variable. For example, we may have scores on tasks like *standing* or *walking with help*.

The *measurement model* specifies the relations between the actual measurements and the latent variable. Under a given measurement model, we may estimate the locations of milestones and children on the line. Section 1.4.5 discusses measurement models in more detail.

1.3.6   WHY UNIT-BASED MEASUREMENT?

This section distinguishes four approaches to measure child development: *age-based*, *probability-based*, *score-based* and *unit-based* measurement. Table 1.3.1 summarizes how the approaches evaluate on nine criteria.

Age-based measurement expresses development in age equivalents, whose precise definition depends on the reference population. Age-based measurement does not support multiple milestones and does not use the concept of a latent variable.

Probability-based measurement expresses development as age percentiles for a reference population. It is useful for individual milestones but does not support multiple items or a latent variable interpretation.

Score-based measurement quantifies development by summing the number of passes. Different instruments make different selections of milestones, so the scores taken are unique to the tool. Thus comparing the measurement obtained by different devices is difficult. Skipping or adding items require corrections.

Unit-based measurement defines a unit by a theoretical model. When the data fit the model, we are able to construct instruments that produce values in a standard metric.

TABLE 1.3.1
Evaluation of four measurement approaches on seven criteria.

Criterion	Age	Probability	Score	Unit
Independent of age norm	No	No	Yes	Yes
Supports multiple milestones	No	No	Yes	Yes
Latent variable	No	No	Yes	Yes
Robust to milestone skipping	Yes	Yes	No	Yes
Comparable scores	Yes	Yes	No	Yes
Probability model	No	Yes	No	Yes
Defines measurement unit	No	No	No	Yes

1.4 The D-score

Stef van Buuren[1,2]
Iris Eekhout[1]
[1]Netherlands Organisation for Applied Scientific
Research TNO, Leiden, 2316 ZL, The Netherlands
[2]University of Utrecht, Utrecht, 3584 CH, The
Netherlands

Section 1.2 provided historical background on the nature of child development. Section 1.3 discussed three general quantification approaches. This section explains how to apply the unit-based approach to arrive at the D-score scale. The text illustrates the process with real data.

- Dutch Development Instrument (DDI) (1.4.1)
- Milestone passing by age and by D-score (1.4.2, 1.4.3)
- How do age and D-score relate? (1.4.4)
- Role of the measurement model (1.4.5)
- Item and person response functions (1.4.6)
- Engelhard invariance criteria (1.4.7)
- Why the Rasch model? (1.4.8)

1.4.1 THE DUTCH DEVELOPMENT INSTRUMENT (DDI)

1.4.1.1 SETTING

The Dutch Youth Health Care (YHC) routinely monitors the development of almost all children living in The Netherlands. During the first four years, there are 13 scheduled visits. During these visits, the YHC professionals evaluate the growth and development of the child.

The *Dutch Development Instrument* (DDI; in Dutch: *Van Wiechenschema*) is the standard instrument used to measure development during the ages 0–4 years. The DDI consists of 75 milestones. The instrument assesses three developmental domains:

1. Fine motor, adaptation, personality and social behaviour;
2. Communication;
3. Gross motor.

The milestones form two sets, one for children aged 0–15 months, and another for children aged 15–54 months. The YHC professionals administer an age-appropriate subset of milestones at each of the scheduled visits, thus building a *longitudinal developmental profile* for each child.

DOI: 10.1201/9781003216315-4

1.4.1.2   Description of SMOCC study

The Social Medical Survey of Children Attending Child Health Clinics (SMOCC) study is a nationally representative cohort of 2,151 children born in The Netherlands during the years 1988–1989 (Herngreen *et al.*, 1994). The study monitored child development using observations made on the DDI during nine visits covering the first 24 months of life. The SMOCC study collected information during the first two years on 57 (out of 75) milestones.

The *standard* set in the DDI consists of relatively easy milestones that 90 per cent of the children can pass at the scheduled age. This set is designed to have maximal sensitivity for picking up delays in development. A distinctive feature of the SMOCC study was the inclusion of more difficult milestones beyond the standard set. The *additional* set originates from the next time point. The success rate on these milestones is about 50 per cent.

1.4.1.3   Codebook of DDI 0–30 months

Table 1.4.1 shows the 57 milestones from the DDI for ages 0 – 30 months as administered in the SMOCC study. Items are sorted according to *debut*, the age at which the item appears in the DDI. The response to each milestone is either a PASS (1) or a FAIL (0). Children who did not pass a milestone at the debut age were re-measured on that milestone during the next visit. The process continued until the child passed the milestone.

1.4.2   PROBABILITY OF PASSING A MILESTONE GIVEN AGE

Figure 1.4.1 summarizes the response obtained on each milestone as a curve against age. The percentage of pass scores increases with age for all milestones. Note that curves on the left have steeper slopes than those on the right, thus indicating that development is faster for younger children.

The domain determines the coloured (blue: gross motor, green: fine motor, red: communication). In general, domains are well mixed across age, though around some ages, e.g., at four months, multiple milestones from the same domain appear.

1.4.3   PROBABILITY OF PASSING A MILESTONE GIVEN D-SCORE

Figure 1.4.2 is similar to Figure 1.4.1, but with the horizontal axis replaced by the D-score. The D-score summarizes development into one number. See 1.5.3 for a detailed explanation on how to calculate the D-score. The vertical axis with per cent pass is unchanged.

The percentage of successes increases with D-score for all milestones. In contrast to Figure 1.4.1 all curves have a similar slope, a desirable property needed for an interval scale with a constant unit of measurement (cf. Section 1.3.4).

TABLE 1.4.1
Codebook of DDI as used in the SMOCC study.

Item	Debut	Domain	Label
ddicmm029	1m	Communication	Reacts when spoken to
ddifmd001	1m	Fine motor	Eyes fixate
ddigmd052	1m	Gross motor	Moves arms equally well
ddigmd053	1m	Gross motor	Moves legs equally well
ddigmd056	1m	Gross motor	Lifts chin off table for a moment
ddicmm030	2m	Communication	Smiles in response (M; can ask parents)
ddifmd002	2m	Fine motor	Follows with eyes and head 30d < 0 > 30d
ddicmm031	3m	Communication	vocalizes in response
ddifmd003	3m	Fine motor	Hands open occasionally
ddifmm004	3m	Fine motor	Watches own hands
ddigmd054	3m	Gross motor	Stays suspended when lifted under the armpits
ddigmd057	3m	Gross motor	Lifts head to 45 degrees on prone position
ddicmd116	6m	Communication	Turn head to sound
ddifmd005	6m	Fine motor	Plays with hands in midline
ddigmd006	6m	Gross motor	Grasps object within reach
ddigmd055	6m	Gross motor	No head lag if pulled to sitting
ddigmd058	6m	Gross motor	Looks around to side with angle face-table 90
ddigmd059	6m	Gross motor	Flexes or stomps legs while being swung
ddicmm033	9m	Communication	Says dada, baba, gaga
ddifmd007	9m	Fine motor	Passes cube from hand to hand
ddifmd008	9m	Fine motor	Holds cube, grasps another one with other hand
ddifmm009	9m	Fine motor	Plays with both feet
ddigmm060	9m	Gross motor	Rolls over back to front
ddigmd061	9m	Gross motor	Balances head well while sitting
ddigmd062	9m	Gross motor	Sits on buttocks while legs stretched
ddicmm034	12m	Communication	Babbles while playing
ddicmm036	12m	Communication	Waves 'bye-bye' (M; can ask parents)
ddifmd010	12m	Fine motor	Picks up pellet between thumb and index finger
ddigmd063	12m	Gross motor	Sits in stable position without support
ddigmm064	12m	Gross motor	Crawls forward, abdomen on the floor
ddigmm065	12m	Gross motor	Pulls up to standing position
ddicmm037	15m	Communication	Uses two words with comprehension
ddicmd136	15m	Communication	Reacts to verbal request (M; can ask parents)
ddifmd011	15m	Fine motor	Puts cube in and out of a box
ddifmm012	15m	Fine motor	Plays 'give and take' (M; can ask parents)
ddigmm066	15m	Gross motor	Crawls, abdomen off the floor (M; can ask parents)
ddigmm067	15m	Gross motor	Walks while holding onto play-pen or furniture
ddicmm039	18m	Communication	Says three 'words'
ddicmd141	18m	Communication	Identifies two named objects
ddifmd013	18m	Fine motor	Tower of 2 cubes

(Continued)

TABLE 1.4.1
(Continued)

Item	Debut	Domain	Label
ddifmm014	18m	Fine motor	Explores environment energetically (M; can ask parents)
ddigmd068	18m	Gross motor	Walks alone
ddigmd069	18m	Gross motor	Throws ball without falling
ddicmm041	24m	Communication	Says sentences with 2 words
ddicmd148	24m	Communication	Understands 'play' orders
ddifmd015	24m	Fine motor	Builds tower of 3 cubes
ddifmm016	24m	Fine motor	Imitates everyday activities (M; can ask parents)
ddigmd070	24m	Gross motor	Squats or bends to pick things up
ddigmd146	24m	Gross motor	Drinks from cup (M; can ask parents)
ddigmd168	24m	Gross motor	Walks well
ddicmm043	30m	Communication	Refers to self using 'me' or 'I' (M; can ask parents)
ddicmd044	30m	Communication	Points at 5 pictures in the book
ddifmd017	30m	Fine motor	Tower of 6 cubes
ddifmd018	30m	Fine motor	Places round block in board
ddifmm019	30m	Fine motor	Takes off shoes and socks (M; can ask parents)
ddifmd154	30m	Fine motor	Eats with spoon without help (M; can ask parents)
ddigmd071	30m	Gross motor	Kicks ball

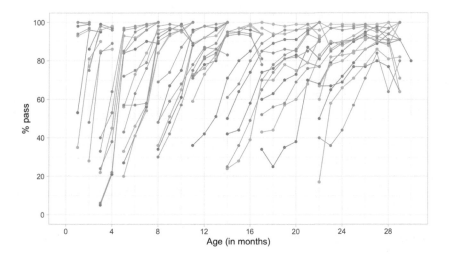

FIGURE 1.4.1 Empirical percentage of passing each milestone in the DDI against age (Source: SMOCC data, $n = 2151$, 9 occasions).

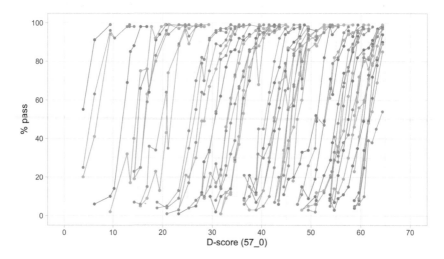

FIGURE 1.4.2 Empirical percentage of passing each milestone in the DDI against the D-score (Source: SMOCC data, 2151 children, 9 occasions).

How can the relation between per cent pass and age be so different from the relation between per cent pass and the D-score? The next section explains the reason.

1.4.4   RELATION BETWEEN AGE AND THE D-SCORE

Figure 1.4.3 shows that the relation between D-score and age is nonlinear. Development in the first year is more rapid than in the second year. During the first year, infants gain about 40 *D*, whereas in the second year they gain about 20 *D*. A similar change in growth rate occurs in length (first year: 23 cm, second year: 12 cm, for Dutch children).

Figure 1.4.4 shows the mutual relations between age, percentage of milestone passing and the D-score. There are three main orientations.

- In the default orientation (age on the horizontal axis, D-score on the vertical axis), we see a curvilinear relation between the age and item difficulty.
- Rotate the graph (age on the horizontal axis, passing percentage on the vertical axis). Observe that this is the same pattern as in Figure 1.4.1 (with *unequal slopes*). Curves are coloured by domain.
- Rotate the graph (D-score on the horizontal axis, passing percentage on the vertical axis). Observe that this pattern is the same as in Figure 1.4.2 (with *equal slopes*).

All patterns can co-exist because of the curvature in the relation between D-score and age. The curvature is never explicitly modelled or defined, but a

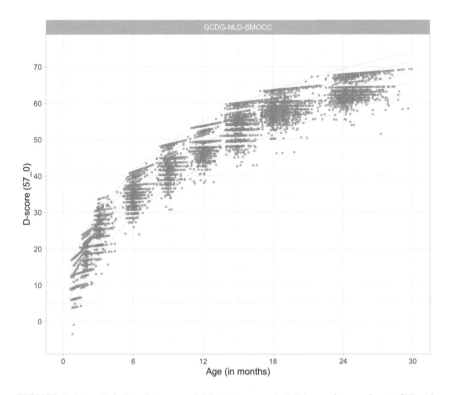

FIGURE 1.4.3 Relation between child D-score and child age in a cohort of Dutch children (Source: SMOCC data, *n* = 2151, 9 occasions).

consequence of the equal-slopes assumption in the relation between the D-score and the passing percentage of a milestone.

1.4.5 MEASUREMENT MODEL FOR THE D-SCORE

1.4.5.1 WHAT ARE MEASUREMENT MODELS?

From section 1.3.5 we quote:

> The measurement model specifies the relations between the data and the latent variable.

The term *Item Response Theory* (IRT) refers to the scientific theory of measurement models. Good introductory works include Embretsen & Reise (2000); Wright & Masters (1982) and Engelhard Jr. (2013).

IRT models enable quantification of the locations of both *items (milestones) and* persons* on the latent variable. We reserve the term *item* for generic properties, and *milestone* for child development. In general, items are part of the measurement instrument, persons are the objects to be measured.

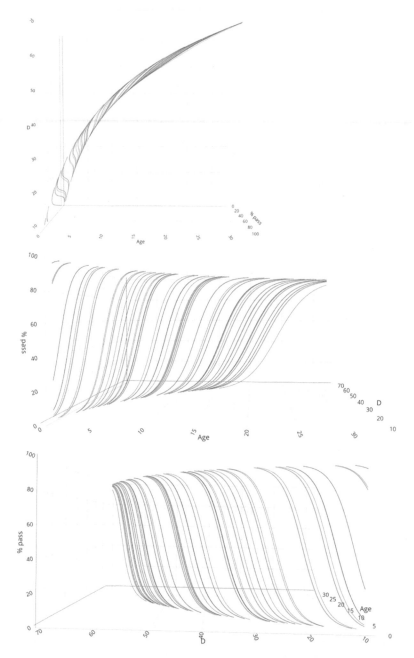

FIGURE 1.4.4   3D-line graph illustrating how the patterns in Figure 1.4.1 and Figure 1.4.2 induce the curvature in the relation between D-score and age.

The printed version shows three orientations of the relation between age, percent pass and D-score. The online version holds an interactive 3D graph that the reader can actively manipulate the orientation of the graph by click-hold-drag mouse operations.

An IRT model has three major structural components:

- Specification of the underlying *latent variable(s)*. In this work, we restrict ourselves to models with just one latent variable. Multi-dimensional IRT models do have their uses, but they are complicated to fit and not widely used;
- For a given item, a specification of the *probability of success* given a value on the latent variables. This specification can take many forms. Section 1.4.6 focuses on this in more detail;
- Specification how probability models for the different items should be combined. In this work, we will restrict to models that assume *local independence* of the probabilities. In that case, the probability of passing two items is equal to the product of success probabilities.

1.4.5.2 ADAPT THE MODEL? OR ADAPT THE DATA?

The measurement model induces a predictable pattern in the observed items. We can test this pattern against the observed data. When there is misfit between the expected and observed data, we can follow two strategies:

- Make the measurement model more general;
- Discard items (and sometimes persons) to make the model fit.

These are very different strategies that have led to heated debates among psychometricians. See Engelhard Jr. (2013) for an overview.

In this work, we opt for the - rigorous - Rasch model (Rasch (1960)) and will adapt the data to reduce discrepancies between model and data. Arguments for this choice are given later, in Section 1.4.8.

1.4.6 ITEM RESPONSE FUNCTIONS

Most measurement models describe the probability of passing an item as a function of the *difference* between the person's ability and the item's difficulty. A person with low ability will almost inevitably fail a heavy item, whereas a highly able person will almost surely pass an easy item.

Let us now introduce a few symbols. We adopt the notation used in Wright & Masters (1982). We use β_n (ability) to refer to the true (but unknown) developmental score of child n. Symbol δ_i (difficulty) is the true (but unknown) difficulty of an item i, and π_{ni} is the probability that child n passes item i. See Appendix A for a complete list.

The difference between the ability of child n and difficulty of item i is

$$\beta_n - \delta_i$$

In the special case that $\beta_n = \delta_i$, the person will have a probability of 0.5 of passing the item.

1.4.6.1 LOGISTIC MODEL

A widely used method is to express differences on the latent scale in terms of *logistic units* (or *logits*) (Berkson, 1944). The reason preferring the logistic over the linear unit is that its output returns a probability value that maps to discrete events. In our case, we can describe the probability of passing an item (milestone) as a function of the difference between β_n and δ_i expressed in logits.

Figure 1.4.5 shows how the percentage of children that pass the item varies in terms of the ability-difficulty gap $\beta_n - \delta_i$. The gap can vary either by β_n or δ_i so that we may use the graph in two ways:

- To find the probability of passing items with various difficulties for a child with ability β_n. If $\delta_i = \beta_n$ then $\pi_{ni} = 0.5$. If $\delta_i < \beta_n$ then $\pi_{ni} > 0.5$, and if $\delta_i > \beta_n$ then $\pi_{ni} < 0.5$. In words: If the difficulty of the item is equal to the child's ability, then the child has a 50/50 chance to pass. The child will have a higher than 50/50 chance of passing for items with lower difficulty and have a lower than 50/50 chance of passing for items with difficulties that exceed the child's ability.
- To find the probability of passing a given item δ_i for children that vary in ability. If $\beta_n < \delta_i$ then $\pi_{ni} < 0.5$, and if $\beta_n > \delta_i$ then $\pi_{ni} > 0.5$. In words: Children with abilities lower than the item's difficulty will have lower than 50/50 chance of passing, whereas children with abilities that exceed the item's difficulty will have a higher than 50/50 chance of passing.

Formula (1.4.1) defines the standard logistic curve:

$$\pi_{ni} = \frac{\exp(\beta_n - \delta_i)}{1 + \exp(\beta_n - \delta_i)}$$

Formula 1.4.1

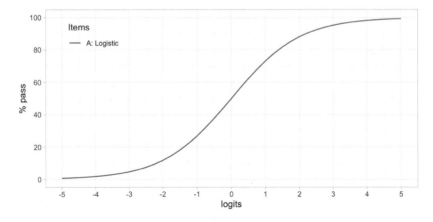

FIGURE 1.4.5 Standard logistic curve. Percentage of children passing an item for a given ability-difficulty gap $\beta_n - \delta_i$.

One way to interpret the formula is as follows. The logarithm of the odds that a person with ability β_n passes an item of difficulty δ_i is equal to the difference $\beta_n-\delta_i$ (Wright & Masters, 1982). For example, suppose that the probability that person n passes milestone i is $\pi_{ni} = 0.5$. In that case, the odds of passing is equal to $0.5/(1 - 0.5) = 1$, so $\log(1) = 0$ and thus $\beta_n = \delta_i$. If $\beta_n-\delta_i = \log(2) = 0.693$ person n is *two* times more likely to pass than to fail. Likewise, if the difference is $\beta_n-\delta_i = \log(3) = 1.1$, then person n is *three* more likely to pass. And so on.

1.4.6.2 TYPES OF ITEM RESPONSE FUNCTIONS

The standard logistic function is by no means the only option to map the relationship between the latent variable and the probability of passing an item. The logistic function is the dominant choice in IRT, but it is instructive to study some other mappings. The *item response function* maps success probability against ability.

Figure 1.4.6 illustrates several other possibilities. Let us consider five hypothetical items, A–E. Note that the horizontal axis now refers to the ability, instead of the ability-item gap in 1.4.5.

- A: Item A is the logistic function discussed in Section 1.4.6.
- B: For item B, the probability of passing is constant at 30 per cent. This 30 per cent is not related to ability. Item B does not measure ability, only adds to the noise, and is of low quality.
- C: Item C is a step function centred at an ability level of 1, so *all* children with an ability below 1 logit fail and *all* children with ability above 1 logit pass. Item C is the ideal item for discriminating children with abilities above and below 1. The item is not sensitive to differences at other ability levels, and often not so realistic in practice.

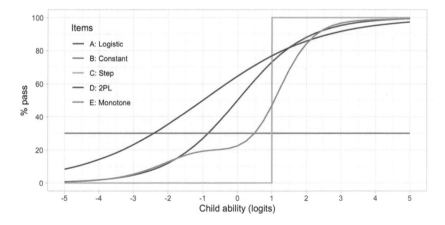

FIGURE 1.4.6 Item response functions for five hypothetical items, each demonstrating a positive relation between ability and probability to pass.

- D: Like A, item D is a smoothly increasing logistic function, but it has an extra parameter that allows it to vary its slope (or discrimination). The extra parameter can make the curve steeper (more discriminatory) than the red curve, in the limit approaching a step curve. It can also become shallower (less discriminatory) than the red curve (as plotted here), in the limit approaching a constant curve (item B). Thus, item D generalizes items A, B or C.
- E: Item E is even more general in the sense that it need not be logistic, but a general monotonically increasing function. As plotted, the item is insensitive to abilities between -1 and 0 logits, and more sensitive to abilities between 0 to 2 logits.

These are just some examples of how the relationship between the child's ability and passing probability could look. In practice, the curves need not start at 0 per cent or end at 100 per cent. They could also be U-shaped, or have other non-monotonic forms. See Coombs (1964) for a thorough overview of such models. In practice, most models are restricted to shapes A-D.

1.4.6.3 PERSON RESPONSE FUNCTIONS

We can reverse the roles of persons and items. The *person response function* tells us how likely it is that a single person can pass an item, or more commonly, a set of items.

Let us continue with items A, C and D from Figure 1.4.6, and calculate the response function for three children, respectively with abilities $\beta_1 = -2$, $\beta_2 = 0$ and $\beta_3 = 2$.

Figure 1.4.7 presents the person response functions from three persons with abilities of -2, 0 and +2 logits. We calculate the functions as the average of

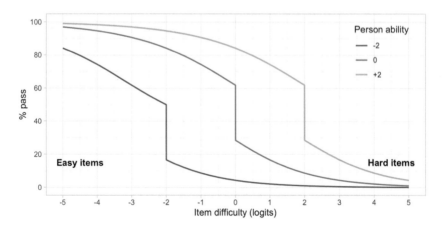

FIGURE 1.4.7   Person response functions for three children with abilities -2, 0 and +2, using a small test of items A, C and D.

response probabilities on items A, C and D. Thus, on average, we expect that child 1 logit will pass an easy item of difficulty -3 in about 60 per cent of the time, whereas for an intermediate item of difficulty of -1 the passing probability would be 10 per cent. For child 3, with higher ability, these probabilities are quite different: 97% and 90%. The substantial drop in the middle of the curve is due to the step function of item A.

1.4.7 ENGELHARD CRITERIA FOR INVARIANT MEASUREMENT

In this work, we strive to achieve *invariant measurement*, a strict form of measurements that is subject to the following requirements (Engelhard Jr., 2013, 14):

1. *Item-invariant measurement of persons*: The measurement of persons must be independent of the particular items used for the measuring.
2. *Non-crossing person response functions*: A more able person must always have a better chance of success on an item that a less able person.
3. *Person-invariant calibration of test items*: The calibration of the items must be independent of the particular persons used for calibration.
4. *Non-crossing item response functions*: Any person must have a better chance of success on an easy item than on a more difficult item.
5. *Unidimensionality*: Items and persons take on values on a *single* latent variable. Under this assumption, the relations between the items are fully explainable by the scores on the latent scale. In practice, the requirement implies that items should measure the same construct. (Hattie, 1985)

Three families of IRT models support invariant measurement:

1. Scalogram model (Guttman, 1950)
2. Rasch model (Andrich, 1978; Rasch, 1960; Wright & Masters, 1982)
3. Mokken scaling model (Mokken, 1971; Molenaar, 1997)

The Guttman and Mokken models yield an ordinal latent scale, while the Rasch model yields an interval scale (with a constant unit).

1.4.8 WHY TAKE THE RASCH MODEL?

- *Invariant measurement*: The Rasch model meets the five Engelhard criteria (cf. Section 1.4.7).
- *Interval scale*: When it fits, the Rasch model provides an interval scale, the de-facto requirement for any numerical comparisons (cf. Section 1.3.4.1).
- *Parsimonious*: The Rasch model has one parameter for each item and one parameter for each person. The Rash model one of the most parsimonious

IRT models, and can easily be applied to thousands of items and millions of persons.

- *Specific objectivity*: Person and item parameters are mathematically separate entities in the Rasch model. In practice, this means that the estimated difference in ability between two persons does not depend on the difficulty of the test. Also, the estimated differences in difficulties between two items do not depend on the abilities in the calibration sample. The property is especially important in the analysis of combined data, where abilities can vary widely between sources. See Rasch (1977) for derivations and examples.
- *Unified model*: The Rasch model unifies distinct traditions in measurement theory. One may derive the Rasch model from
  - Thorndike's 1904 criteria
  - Guttman scalogram model
  - Ratio-scale counts
  - Raw scores as sufficient statistics
  - Thurstone's scaling requirements
  - Campbell concatenation
  - Rasch's specific objectivity

- *Fits child development data*: Last but not least, as we will see in Section 1.6, the Rasch model provides an excellent fit to child development milestones.

Note that the Rasch model is not unique in all aspects. A reviewer indicated that specific objectivity and invariant measurement might also be achieved in certain 2PL models. For us, the combination of simplicity, interpretability, and convenient properties makes the Rasch model stand out.

1.5 Computation

Stef van Buuren[1,2]
Iris Eekhout[1]
[1]Netherlands Organisation for Applied Scientific
Research TNO, Leiden, 2316 ZL, The Netherlands
[2]University of Utrecht, Utrecht, 3584 CH, The
Netherlands

This section explains the basic computations needed for fitting and evaluating the Rasch model. We distinguish the following steps:

- Identify nature of the problem (1.5.1)
- Estimation of item parameters (1.5.2)
- Anchoring (1.5.2.2)
- Estimation of the D-score (1.5.3)
- Estimation of age-conditional references (1.5.4)

Readers not interested in these details may continue to model evaluation in Section 1.6.

1.5.1 IDENTIFY NATURE OF THE PROBLEM

The SMOCC dataset, introduced in Section 1.4.1.2, contains scores on the DDI of Dutch children aged 0–2 years made during nine visits.

Table 1.5.1 contains data of three children, measured on nine visits between ages 0 – 2 years. The DDI scores take values 0 (FAIL) and 1 (PASS). In order to save horizontal space, we truncated the column headers to the last two digits of the item names.

Since the selection of milestones depends on age, the dataset contains a large number of empty cells. Naive use of sum scores as a proxy to ability is therefore problematic. An empty cell is not a FAIL, so it is incorrect to impute those cells by zeroes.

Note that some rows contain only 1's, e.g., in row 2. Many computer programs for Rasch analysis routinely remove such *perfect scores* before fitting. However, unless the number of perfect scores is very small, this is not recommended because doing so can severely affect the ability distribution.

In order to effectively handle the missing data and to preserve all persons in the analysis we separate estimation of item difficulties (cf. Section 1.5.2) and person abilities (cf. Section 1.5.3).

DOI: 10.1201/9781003216315-5

TABLE 1.5.1
SMOCC DDI milestones, first three children, 0–2 years.

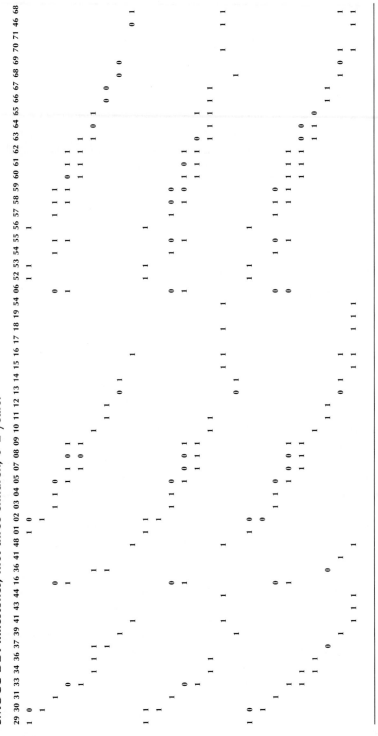

1.5.2   ITEM PARAMETER ESTIMATION

1.5.2.1   PAIRWISE ESTIMATION OF ITEM DIFFICULTIES

There are many methods for estimating the difficulty parameters of the Rasch estimation. See Linacre (2004) for an overview.

We will use the pairwise estimation method. This method writes the probability that child n passes item i but not item j given that the child passed one of them as $\exp(\delta_i)/(\exp(\delta_i) + \exp(\delta_j))$. The method optimizes the pseudo-likelihood of all item pairs over the difficulty estimates by a simple iterative procedure.

Zwinderman (1995) has shown that this procedure provides consistent estimates with similar efficiency as computationally more-intensive conditional and marginal maximum likelihood methods.

The beauty of the method is that it is independent of the ability distribution, so there is no need to remove perfect scores. We use the function `rasch. pairwise.itemcluster()` as implemented in the `sirt` package (Robitzsch, 2016).

Figure 1.5.1 summarizes the estimated item difficulty parameters. Although the model makes no distinction between domains, the results have been ordered to ease spotting of the natural progression of the milestones per domain. The figure also suggests that not all domain have equal representation across the scale. For example, there are no communication milestones around the logit of –10.

1.5.2.2   ANCHORING

The Rasch model identifies the item difficulties up to a linear transformation. By default, the software produces estimates in the logit scale (cf. Figure 1.5.1). The logit scale is inconvenient for two reasons:

- The logit scale has negative values. Negative values do not have a sensible interpretation in child development, and are likely to introduce errors in practice;
- Both the zero in the logit scale, as well as its variance, depend on the sample used to calibrate the item difficulties.

Rescaling preserves the properties of the Rasch model. To make the scale independent of the specified sample, we transform the scale so that two items will always have the same value on the transformed scale. The choice of the two anchor items is essentially arbitrary, but they should correspond to milestones that are easy to measure with small error. In the sequel, we use the two milestones to anchor the D-score scale by the items in Table 1.5.2. With the choice of Table 1.5.2, D-score values are approximately 0 D around birth. At the age of 1 year, the score will around 50 D, so during the first year of life, one D unit corresponds to approximately a one-week interval. Figure 1.5.2 shows the difficulty estimates in the D-score scale.

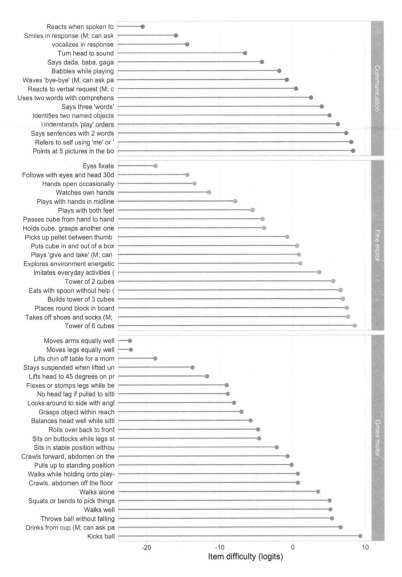

FIGURE 1.5.1 Estimated item difficulty parameters (d_i) for 57 milestones of the DDI
(0 – 2 years).

TABLE 1.5.2

Anchoring values used to identify the D-score scale.

Item	Label	Value
ddigmd057	Lifts head to 45 degrees on prone position	20
ddigmd063	Sits in stable position without support	40

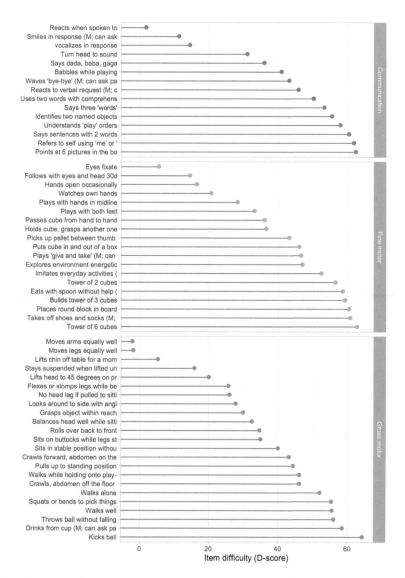

FIGURE 1.5.2 Estimated item difficulty parameters (d_i) for 57 milestones of the DDI (0 – 2 years).

Milestones `ddigmd057` and `ddigmd063` are anchored at values of 20 D and 40 D, respectively.

1.5.3 ESTIMATION OF THE D-SCORE

The second part of the estimation process is to estimate a D-score. The D-score quantifies the development of a child at a given age. Whereas the instrument developer is responsible for the estimation of item parameters, D-score estimation is more of a task for the user. To calculate the D-score, we need the following ingredients:

- Child's PASS/FAIL scores on the milestones administered;
- The difficulty estimates of each milestone administered;
- A prior distribution, an estimate of the D-score distribution before seeing any PASS/FAIL score.

Using these inputs, we may use Bayes theorem to calculate the position of the person on the latent variable.

1.5.3.1 ROLE OF THE STARTING PRIOR

The first two inputs to the D-score will be self-evident. The third component, the prior distribution, is needed to be able to deal with perfect responses. The prior distribution summarizes our knowledge about the D-score before we see any of the child's PASS/FAIL scores. In general, we like the prior to be non-informative, so that the observed responses and item difficulties entirely determine the value of the D-score. In practice, we cannot use truly non-informative prior because that would leave the D-score for perfect responses (i.e., all PASS or all FAIL) undefined. The choice of the prior is essentially arbitrary, but we can make it in such a way that its impact on the value D-score is negligible, especially for tests where we have more than, say, four items.

Since we know that the D-score depends on age, a logical choice for the prior is to make it dependent on age. In particular, we will define the prior as a normal distribution equal to the expected mean in Figure 1.4.3 at the child's age, and with a standard deviation that considerably higher than in Figure 1.4.3. Numerical example: the mean D-score at the age of 15 months is equal to 53.6 D. The standard deviation in Figure 1.4.3 varies between 2.6 D and 3.0 D, with an average of 2.9 D. After some experimentation, we found that using a value of 5.0 D for the prior yields a good compromise between non-informativeness and robustness of D-score estimates for perfect patterns. The resulting starting prior for a child aged 15 months is thus $N(53.6,5)$.

The reader now probably wonders about a chicken-and-egg problem: To calculate the D-score, we need a prior, and to determine the prior we need the D-score. So how did we calculate the D-scores in Figure 1.4.3? The answer is that we first took at rougher prior, and calculated two temporary models in succession using the D-scores obtained after solution 1 to inform the prior before solution 2, and so on. It turned out that D-scores in Figure 1.4.3 hardly changed after two steps, and so there we stopped.

1.5.3.2 STARTING PRIOR: NUMERICAL EXAMPLE

Figure 1.5.3 illustrates starting distributions (priors) chosen according to the principles set above for the ages of 1, 15 and 24 months. As expected, the assumed ability of an infant aged one month is much lower than that of a child aged 15 months, which in turn is lower than the ability of a toddler aged 24 months. The green distribution for 15 months corresponds to the normal distribution N (53.6,5).

Another choice that we need to make is the grid of points on which we calculate the prior and posterior distributions. Figure 1.5.3 uses a grid from -10 D to +80 D, with a step size of 1 D. These are fixed *quadrature points*, and there are 91 of them. While these quadrature points are sufficient to estimate D-score for ages up to 2.5 years, it is wise to extend the range for older children with higher D-scores.

1.5.3.3   EAP ALGORITHM

The algorithm for estimating the D-score is known as the Expected a posteriori (EAP) method, first described by Bock & Mislevy (1982). Calculation of the D-score proceeds item by item. Suppose we have some vague and preliminary idea about the distribution of D, the starting prior (cf. section 1.5.3.1), based on age. The procedure uses Bayes rule to update this prior knowledge with data from the first item (using the child's FAIL/PASS score and the estimated item difficulty) to calculate the posterior. The next step uses this posterior as prior before processing the next item, and so on. The procedure stops when the item pool is exhausted. The order in which items enter does not matter for the result. The D-score is equal to the mean of the posterior calculated after the last question.

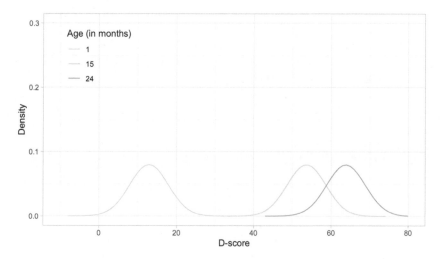

FIGURE 1.5.3   Age-dependent starting priors for the D-score at the ages of 1, 15 and 24 months.

1.5.3.4   EAP ALGORITHM: NUMERICAL EXAMPLE

Suppose we measure two boys aged 15 months, David and Rob, by the DDI. David passes the first four milestones but does not complete the test. Rob completes the test but fails on two out of five items.

Table 1.5.3 shows the difficulty of each milestone (in the column labelled "Delta"), and the responses of David and Rob for the standard five DDI milestones for the age of 15 months.

The mean D-score for Dutch children aged 15 months is 53.6 D, so the milestones are easy to pass at this age, with the most difficult is ddicmm037. David passed all milestones but has no score on the last. Rob fails on ddifmm012 and ddigmm067. How do we calculate the D-score for David and Rob?

Figure 1.5.4 shows how the prior transforms into the posterior after we successively feed the measurements into the calculation. There are five milestones, so the calculation comprises five steps:

1. Both David and Rob pass ddifmd011. The prior (light green) is the same as in Figure 1.5.3. After a PASS, the posterior will be located more to the right, and will often be more peaked. Both happen here, but the change is small. The reason is that a PASS on this milestone is not very informative. For a child with a true D-score of 53 D, the probability of passing ddifmd011 is equal to 0.966. If passing is so common, there is not much information in the measurement.
2. David passes ddifmm012, but Rob does not. Observe that the prior is identical to the posterior of ddifmd011. For David, the posterior is only slightly different from the prior, for the same reason as above. For Rob, we find a considerable change to the left, both for location (from 54.3 D to 47.1 D) and peakedness. This one FAIL lowers Rob's score by 7.2 D.
3. Milestone ddicmm037 is more difficult than the previous two milestones, so a pass on ddicmm037 does have a definite effect on the posterior for both David and Rob.

TABLE 1.5.3
Scores of David and Rob on five milestones from the DDI.

Item	Label	Delta	David	Rob
ddifmd011	Puts cube in and out of a box	46.0	1	1
ddifmm012	Plays "give and take" (M; can ask parents)	46.5	1	0
ddicmm037	Uses two words with comprehension	50.1	1	1
ddigmm066	Crawls, abdomen off the floor (M; can ask parents)	46.1	1	1
ddigmm067	Walks while holding onto play-pen or furniture	46.1		0

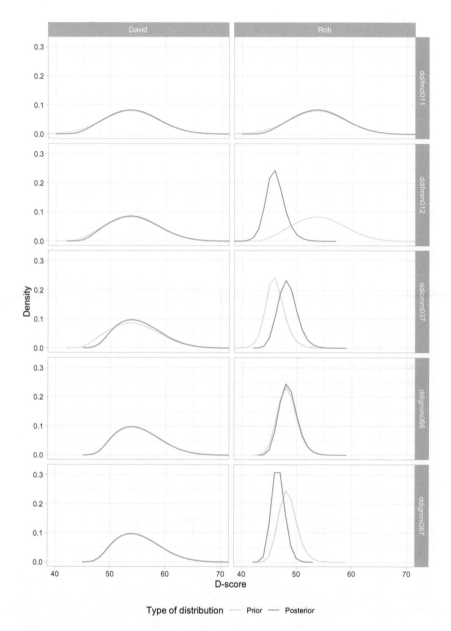

FIGURE 1.5.4 D-score distribution for David and Rob before (prior) and after (posterior) a milestone is taken into account.

4. David's PASS on `ddigmm066` does not bring any additional information, so his prior and posterior are virtually indistinguishable. For Rob, we find a slight shift to the right.
5. There is no measurement for David on `ddigmm067`, so the prior and posterior are equivalent. For Rob, we observe a FAIL, which shifts his posterior to the left.

We calculate the D-score as the mean of the posterior. David's D-score is equal to 55.7 D. Note that the measurement error, as estimated from the variance of the posterior, is relatively large. Rob's D-score is equal to 47.7 D, with a much smaller measurement error. This result is consistent with the design principles of the DDI, which is meant to detect children with developmental delay.

The example illustrates that the quality of the D-score depends on two factors, the match between the true (but unknown) D-score of the child and the difficulty of the milestone.

1.5.3.5 TECHNICAL OBSERVATIONS ON D-SCORE ESTIMATION

- Administration of a too easy set of milestones introduces a *ceiling* with children that pass all milestones, but whose true D-score could extend well beyond the maximum. Depending on the goal of the measurement, this may or may not be a problem.
- The specification of the prior and posterior distributions requires a set of quadrature points. The quadrature points are taken here as the static and evenly-spaced set of integers between -10 and +80. Using other quadrature points may affect the estimate, especially if the range of the quadrature points does not cover the entire D-score range.
- The actual calculations are here done item by item. A more efficient method is to handle all responses at once. The result will be the same.

1.5.4   AGE-CONDITIONAL REFERENCES

1.5.4.1   MOTIVATION

The last step involves estimation an age-conditional reference distribution for the D-score. This distribution can be used to construct growth charts that portray the normal variation in development. Also, the references can be used to calculate age-standardized D-scores, called DAZ, that emphasize the location of the measurement in comparison to age peers.

Estimation of reference centiles is reasonably standard. Here we follow van Buuren (2014) to fit age-conditional references of the D-score for boys and girls combined by the LMS method. The LMS method by Cole & Green (1992) assumes that the outcome has a normal distribution after a Box-Cox transformation. The reference distribution has three parameters, which model respectively the location (M), the spread (S), and the skewness (L) of the distribution. Each of the three parameters can vary smoothly with age.

1.5.4.2 ESTIMATION OF THE REFERENCE DISTRIBUTION

The parameters are estimated using the BCCG distribution of `gamlss 5.1-3` (Stasinopoulos & Rigby, 2008) using cubic splines smoothers. The final solution used a log-transformed age scale and fitted the model with smoothing parameters df(M) = 2, df(S) = 2 and df(L) = 1.

Figure 1.4.3 plots the D-scores together with five grey lines, corresponding to the centiles -2SD (P2), -1SD (P16), 0SD (P50), +1SD (P84) and +2SD (P98). The area between the -2SD and +2SD lines delineates the D-score expected if development is healthy. Note that the shape of the reference is quite similar to that of weight and height, with rapid growth occurring in the first few months.

Table 1.5.4 defines age-conditional references for Dutch children as the M-curve (median), S-curve (spread) and L-curve (skewness) by age. This table can be used to calculate centile lines and Z-scores.

The references are purely cross-sectional and do not account for the correlation structure between ages. For prediction purposes, it is useful to extend the modelling to include velocities and change scores.

1.5.4.3 CONVERSION OF D TO DAZ, AND VICE VERSA

Suppose that M_t, S_t and L_t are the parameter values at age t. Cole (1988) shows that the transformation

$$Z = \frac{(D_t/M_t)^{L_t} - 1}{L_t S_t}$$

converts measurement D_t into its normal equivalent deviate Z. If L_t is close to zero, we use

$$Z = \frac{\ln(D_t/M_t)}{S_t}$$

We may derive any required centile curve from Table 1.5.4. First, choose Z_α as the Z-score that delineates 100 α per cent of the distribution, for example, $Z_{0.05} = -1.64$. The D-score that defines the 100 α centile is equal to

$$D_t(\alpha) = M_t(1 + L_t S_t Z_\alpha)^{1/L_t}$$

If L_t is close to zero, we use

$$D_t(\alpha) = M_t \exp(S_t Z_\alpha).$$

TABLE 1.5.4

Dutch reference values for the D-score.

Age	M	S	L
0.0383	8.81	0.3126	1.3917
0.0575	10.59	0.2801	1.4418
0.0767	12.27	0.2526	1.4891
0.0958	13.87	0.2291	1.5331
0.1150	15.39	0.2089	1.5722
0.1342	16.83	0.1916	1.6049
0.1533	18.20	0.1767	1.6304
0.1725	19.50	0.1640	1.6487
0.1916	20.75	0.1531	1.6607
0.2108	21.94	0.1436	1.6676
0.2300	23.07	0.1354	1.6706
0.2491	24.16	0.1283	1.6711
0.2683	25.21	0.1220	1.6698
0.2875	26.21	0.1165	1.6673
0.3066	27.17	0.1117	1.6636
0.3258	28.10	0.1074	1.6589
0.3450	28.99	0.1035	1.6533
0.3641	29.86	0.1001	1.6471
0.3833	30.70	0.0970	1.6403
0.4025	31.50	0.0942	1.6330
0.4216	32.29	0.0917	1.6255
0.4408	33.05	0.0894	1.6178
0.4600	33.79	0.0873	1.6100
0.4791	34.51	0.0854	1.6022
0.4983	35.21	0.0837	1.5946
0.5175	35.89	0.0821	1.5870
0.5366	36.55	0.0807	1.5797
0.5558	37.20	0.0793	1.5725
0.5749	37.83	0.0781	1.5656
0.5941	38.44	0.0770	1.5588
0.6133	39.04	0.0759	1.5523
0.6324	39.63	0.0749	1.5460
0.6516	40.21	0.0740	1.5399
0.6708	40.77	0.0731	1.5340
0.6899	41.32	0.0723	1.5284
0.7091	41.86	0.0715	1.5230
0.7283	42.39	0.0707	1.5178
0.7474	42.91	0.0700	1.5128
0.7666	43.42	0.0693	1.5081
0.7858	43.92	0.0687	1.5036

(Continued)

TABLE 1.5.4
(Continued)

Age	M	S	L
0.8049	44.40	0.0681	1.4993
0.8241	44.88	0.0674	1.4952
0.8433	45.36	0.0669	1.4913
0.8624	45.82	0.0663	1.4876
0.8816	46.27	0.0657	1.4841
0.9008	46.72	0.0652	1.4809
0.9199	47.16	0.0647	1.4778
0.9391	47.59	0.0642	1.4749
0.9582	48.01	0.0637	1.4723
0.9774	48.43	0.0632	1.4698
0.9966	48.84	0.0627	1.4676
1.0157	49.24	0.0622	1.4655
1.0349	49.64	0.0618	1.4637
1.0541	50.03	0.0613	1.4620
1.0732	50.41	0.0608	1.4605
1.0924	50.79	0.0604	1.4592
1.1116	51.16	0.0600	1.4580
1.1307	51.53	0.0595	1.4570
1.1499	51.89	0.0591	1.4561
1.1691	52.24	0.0587	1.4553
1.1882	52.59	0.0583	1.4547
1.2074	52.94	0.0578	1.4542
1.2266	53.27	0.0574	1.4538
1.2457	53.61	0.0570	1.4535
1.2649	53.94	0.0566	1.4534
1.2841	54.26	0.0562	1.4533
1.3032	54.58	0.0559	1.4533
1.3224	54.89	0.0555	1.4533
1.3415	55.20	0.0551	1.4535
1.3607	55.50	0.0547	1.4537
1.3799	55.81	0.0544	1.4539
1.3990	56.10	0.0540	1.4542
1.4182	56.39	0.0536	1.4546
1.4374	56.68	0.0533	1.4551
1.4565	56.97	0.0530	1.4555
1.4757	57.25	0.0526	1.4561
1.4949	57.52	0.0523	1.4567
1.5140	57.80	0.0520	1.4573
1.5332	58.06	0.0517	1.4580
1.5524	58.33	0.0514	1.4587

(Continued)

TABLE 1.5.4
(Continued)

Age	M	S	L
1.5715	58.59	0.0510	1.4595
1.5907	58.85	0.0508	1.4603
1.6099	59.11	0.0505	1.4612
1.6290	59.36	0.0502	1.4620
1.6482	59.61	0.0499	1.4630
1.6674	59.86	0.0496	1.4639
1.6865	60.11	0.0494	1.4649
1.7057	60.35	0.0491	1.4660
1.7248	60.59	0.0488	1.4670
1.7440	60.82	0.0486	1.4681
1.7632	61.06	0.0483	1.4692
1.7823	61.29	0.0481	1.4704
1.8015	61.52	0.0478	1.4716
1.8207	61.75	0.0476	1.4728
1.8398	61.97	0.0474	1.4740
1.8590	62.20	0.0471	1.4752
1.8782	62.42	0.0469	1.4765
1.8973	62.64	0.0467	1.4778
1.9165	62.85	0.0465	1.4791
1.9357	63.07	0.0463	1.4805
1.9548	63.28	0.0461	1.4818
1.9740	63.49	0.0459	1.4832
1.9932	63.70	0.0457	1.4846
2.0123	63.91	0.0455	1.4861
2.0315	64.11	0.0453	1.4875
2.0507	64.32	0.0451	1.4890
2.0698	64.52	0.0449	1.4904
2.0890	64.72	0.0447	1.4919
2.1081	64.92	0.0445	1.4934
2.1273	65.11	0.0443	1.4949
2.1465	65.31	0.0441	1.4964
2.1656	65.50	0.0440	1.4979
2.1848	65.70	0.0438	1.4994
2.2040	65.89	0.0436	1.5009
2.2231	66.08	0.0434	1.5024
2.2423	66.26	0.0433	1.5039
2.2615	66.45	0.0431	1.5054
2.2806	66.64	0.0429	1.5069
2.2998	66.82	0.0428	1.5084
2.3190	67.00	0.0426	1.5098

(Continued)

TABLE 1.5.4
(Continued)

Age	M	S	L
2.3381	67.18	0.0425	1.5113
2.3573	67.36	0.0423	1.5127
2.3765	67.54	0.0421	1.5142
2.3956	67.72	0.0420	1.5156
2.4148	67.89	0.0418	1.5170
2.4339	68.07	0.0417	1.5185
2.4531	68.24	0.0415	1.5199
2.4723	68.41	0.0414	1.5213
2.4914	68.59	0.0412	1.5226
2.5106	68.75	0.0411	1.5240
2.5298	68.92	0.0410	1.5254
2.5489	69.09	0.0408	1.5267
2.5681	69.26	0.0407	1.5281
2.5873	69.42	0.0405	1.5294
2.6064	69.59	0.0404	1.5308
2.6256	69.75	0.0403	1.5321
2.6448	69.91	0.0401	1.5334
2.6639	70.07	0.0400	1.5347
2.6831	70.23	0.0399	1.5360
2.7023	70.39	0.0397	1.5373
2.7214	70.55	0.0396	1.5386
2.7406	70.71	0.0395	1.5398
2.7598	70.86	0.0394	1.5411
2.7789	71.02	0.0392	1.5423

1.6 Evaluation

Stef van Buuren[1,2]
Iris Eekhout[1]
[1]Netherlands Organisation for Applied Scientific
Research TNO, Leiden, 2316 ZL, The Netherlands
[2]University of Utrecht, Utrecht, 3584 CH, The
Netherlands

The properties cut-off Rasch model (cf. Section 1.4.8) only hold when the data and model agree. It is, therefore, essential to study and remove discrepancies between model and data. This section explains several techniques that aid in the evaluation of model fit.

- Item fit (1.6.1)
- Person fit (1.6.2)
- Differential item functioning (1.6.3)
- Item information (1.6.4)
- Reliability (1.6.5)

These topics address different aspects of the solution. In practice, we have found that item fit is the most critical concern.

1.6.1 ITEM FIT

The philosophy of the Rasch model is different from conventional statistical modelling. It is not the task of the Rasch model to account for the data. Rather it is the task of the data to fit the Rasch model. We saw this distinction before in Section 1.4.5.2.

The goal of model-fit assessment is to explore and quantify how well empirical data meet the requirements of the Rasch model. One way to gauge model-fit is to compare the observed probability of passing an item to the fitted item response curve for endorsing the item.

The fitted item response curve for each item i is modelled as:

$$P_{ni} = \frac{\exp(\widehat{\beta}_n - \widehat{\delta}_i)}{1 + \exp(\widehat{\beta}_n - \widehat{\delta}_i)},$$

where $\widehat{\beta}_n$ is the estimated ability of child n (the child's D-score), and where $\widehat{\delta}_i$ is the estimated difficulty of item i. This is equivalent to formula (1.4.1) with the parameters replaced by estimates. Section 1.5 described process of parameter estimation in some detail.

DOI: 10.1201/9781003216315-6

1.6.1.1   WELL-FITTING ITEM RESPONSE CURVES

The study of *item fit* involves comparing the empirical and fitted probabilities at various levels of ability. Figure 1.6.1 shows the item characteristics curves of two DDI milestones. The orange line represents the empirical probability at different ability levels. The dashed line represents the estimated item response curve according to the Rasch model. The observed and estimated curves are close together, so both items fit the model very well.

1.6.1.2   ITEM RESPONSE CURVES SHOWING SEVERE UNDERFIT

There are many cases where things are less bright.

Figure 1.6.2 shows three forms of severe underfit from three artificial items. These items were simulated to have a low fit, added to the DDI, and we estimated their parameters by the methods of Section 1.5. For the first item,

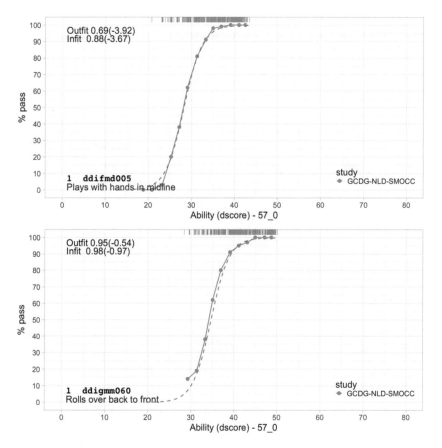

FIGURE 1.6.1   Empirical and fitted item response curves for two milestones from the DDI (SMOCC data).

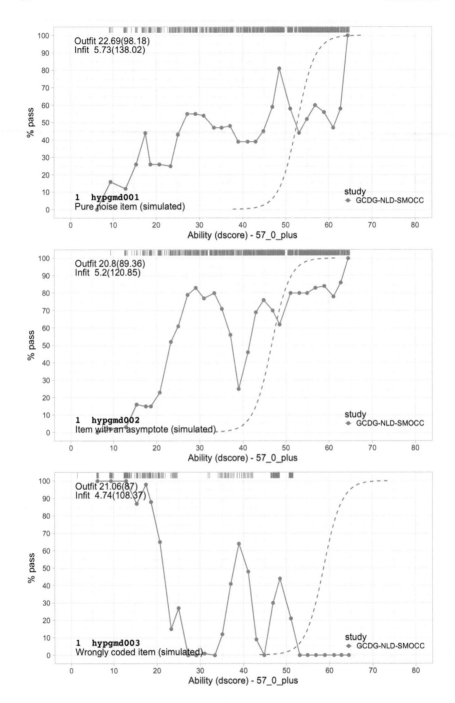

FIGURE 1.6.2 Three simulated items that illustrate various forms of item misfit.

`hypgmd001`, the probability of passing is almost constant across ability, so retaining this item essentially only adds to the noise. Item `hypgmd002` converges to an asymptote around 80 per cent and has a severe dip in the middle. The strong relation to age causes the drop. Item `hypgmd003` appears to have the wrong coding. Also, we often see the spike-like behaviour in the middle when two or more different items erroneously share identical names.

Removal of items with a low fit can substantially improve overall model fit.

1.6.1.3 ITEM RESPONSE CURVES SHOWING OVERFIT

Figure 1.6.3 shows two artificial items with two forms of overfitting. The curve of item `hypgmd004` is much steeper than the modelled curve. Thus, just this one item is exceptionally well-suited to distinguish children with a D-score below 50 D from those with a score above 50 D. Note that the item isn't sensitive anywhere else on the scale. In general, having items like these is good news, because they allow us to increase the reliability of the instrument. One

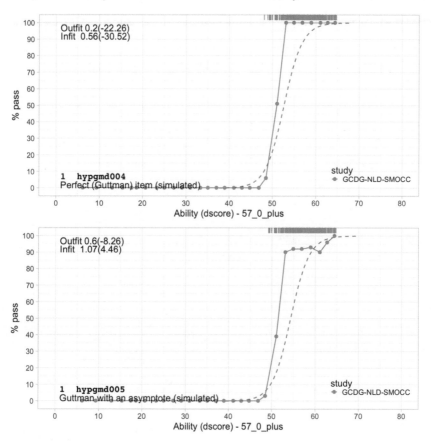

FIGURE 1.6.3 Two simulated items that illustrate item overfit.

should make sure, though, that FAIL and PASS scores are all measured (not imputed) values.

Multiple perfect items could hint to a violation of the *local independence assumption* (cf. Section 1.4.5). Developmental milestones sometimes have combinations of responses that are impossible. For example, one cannot walk without being able to stand, so we will not observe the inconsistent combination (stand: FAIL, walk: PASS). This impossibility leads to more consistent responses that would be expected by chance alone. In principle, one could combine the two such items into one three-category item, which effectively set the probability of inconsistent combinations to zero.

Item `hypgmd005` is also steep, but has an asymptote around 80 per cent. This tail behaviour causes discrepancies between the empirical and modelled curves around the middle of the probability scale. In general, we may remove such items if a sufficient number of alternatives is available.

1.6.1.4 ITEM INFIT AND OUTFIT

We quantify item fit by item *infit* and *outfit*. Both are aggregates of the model residuals. The observed response x_{ni} of person n on item i can be 0 or 1.

The *standardized residual* z_{ni} is the difference between the observed response x_{ni} and the expected response p_{ni}, divided by the expected binomial standard deviation,

$$z_{ni} = \frac{x_{ni} - P_{ni}}{\sqrt{W_{ni}}},$$

where the expected response variance W_{ni} is calculated as

$$W_{ni} = P_{ni}(1 - P_{ni}).$$

Item infit is the total of the squared residuals divided by the sum of the expected response variances W_{ni}

$$\text{Item infit} = \frac{\sum_n^N (x_{ni} - P_{ni})^2}{\sum_n^N W_{ni}}.$$

Item outfit is calculated as the average (over N measurements) of the squared standardized residual

$$\text{Item outfit} = \frac{\sum_n^N z_{ni}^2}{N}.$$

The expected value of both infit and outfit is equal to 1.0. The interpretation is as follows:

- If infit and outfit are 1.0, then the item perfectly fits the Rasch model, as in Figure 1.6.1;
- If infit and outfit > 1.0, then the item is not fitting well. The amount of underfit is quantified by infit and outfit, as in 1.6.2;
- If infit and outfit < 1.0, then the item fits the model better than expected (overfit). Overfitting is quantified by infit and outfit, as in 1.6.3.

Infit is more sensitive to disparities in the middle of the probability scale, whereas outfit is the better measure for discrepancies at probabilities close to 0 or 1. Lack of fit is generally easier to spot at the extremes. The two measures are highly correlated. Achieving good infit is more valuable than a high outfit.

Values near 1.0 are desirable. There is no cut and dried cut-off value for infit and outfit. In general, we want to remove underfitting items with infit or outfit values higher than, say, 1.3. Overfitting items (with values lower than 1.0) are not harmful. Preserving these items may help to increase the reliability of the scale. The cut-off chosen also depends on the number of available items. When there are many items to choose from, we could use a stricter criterion, say infit and outfit < 1.0 to select only the absolute best items.

1.6.1.5 INFIT AND OUTFIT IN THE DDI

Figure 1.6.4 displays the histogram of the 57 milestones from the DDI (cf. Section 1.4.1). Most infit values are within the range 0.6 - 1.1.1, thus indicating excellent fit. The two milestones with shallow infit values are ddigmd052 and ddigmd053. These two items screen for paralysis for newborns, so the data contain hardly any fails on these milestones. The outfit statistics also indicate a good fit.

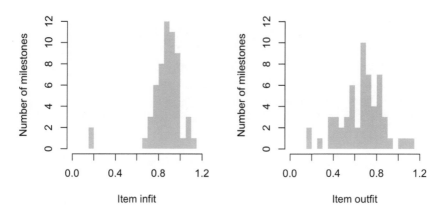

FIGURE 1.6.4 Frequency distribution of infit (left) and outfit (right) of 57 milestones from the DDI (SMOCC data).

1.6.2 PERSON FIT

Person fit quantifies the extent to which the responses of a given child conform to the Rasch model expectation. The Rasch model expects that a more able child has a higher probability of passing an item than a less developed child. Person fit analysis evaluates the extent to which this is true.

1.6.2.1 PERSON INFIT AND OUTFIT

In parallel to item fit, we can calculate *person infit* and *person outfit*. Both statistics evaluate how well the responses of the persons are consistent with the model. Outlying answers that do not fit the expected pattern increase the outfit statistic. The outfit is high, for example, when the child fails easy items but passes difficult ones. The infit is the information weighted fit and is more sensitive to inlaying, on-target, unexpected responses.

Similar to item fit, person fit is also calculated from the residuals, but aggregated differently. We calculate person infit as

$$\text{Person infit} = \frac{\sum_i^L (x_{ni} - P_{ni})^2}{\sum_i^L W_{ni}}$$

and person outfit as

$$\text{Person outfit} = \frac{\sum_i^L z_{ni}^2}{L}$$

A threshold for person fit > 3.0 is customary to clean out children with implausible response patterns.

1.6.2.2 PERSON INFIT AND OUTFIT IN THE DDI

Figure 1.6.5 displays the frequency distribution of person infit and person outfit 16538 measurements of the DDI in the SMOCC data. The majority of the values falls below 3.0. For infit, only 43 out of 16538 fit values (0.3 per cent) is above 3.0. There are 446 out of 16538 outfit value (2.7 per cent) above 3.0. Expect the solution to improve after deleting these measurements.

1.6.3 DIFFERENTIAL ITEM FUNCTIONING (DIF)

1.6.3.1 RELEVANCE OF DIF FOR CROSS-CULTURAL EQUIVALENCE

An essential assumption in the Rasch model is that a given item has the same difficulty in different subgroups of respondents. Climbing stairs is an example where this assumption is suspect. The exposure to stairs, and hence the opportunity for a child to practice, varies across different cultures. It could

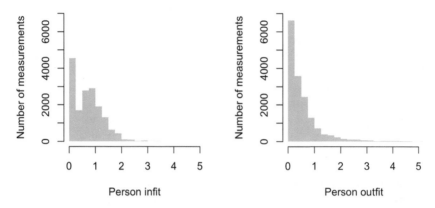

FIGURE 1.6.5   Frequency distribution of person infit (left) and person outfit (right) for 16538 measurements of the DDI (SMOCC data).

thus be that two children with the same ability but from different cultures have different success probabilities for climbing stairs. When these probabilities systematically vary between subgroup, we say there is *Differential Item Functioning*, or *DIF* (Holland & Wainer, 1983). DIF is undesirable since it can make the instrument culturally biased.

1.6.3.2   HOW TO DETECT DIF?

Zumbo (1999) provided a clear definition of DIF:

> DIF occurs when examinees from different groups show differing probabilities of success on (or endorsing) the item after matching on the underlying ability that the item is intended to measure.

There are various ways to detect DIF. Here we will model the probability of endorsing an item by logistic regression using the observed item responses as the outcome. Predictors include the ability, the grouping variable, and the ability-grouping interaction. If the latter two terms explain the residual variance of the item scores after adjusting for ability, the item shows DIF for that group. DIF can be visually inspected by plotting the curves for the subgroups separately.

There are two forms of DIF:

- *Uniform DIF*: The item response curves differ between groups in location, but are parallel;
- *Non-uniform DIF*: The item response curve differ between groups in location, in slope and possibly in other characteristics.

These forms correspond to, respectively, the main effect of group and the ability-group interaction in the logistic regression model.

1.6.3.3 EXAMPLES OF DIF

Figure 1.6.6 shows an example comparing boys and girls. For both milestones, the item response curves are similar for boys and girls, so we see no evidence of DIF here.

Figure 1.6.7 displays two milestones with DIF between boys and girls. Provided that the ability estimate (as estimated from all items in the model) is fair for both boys and girls, we see that milestone ddifmm019 ("Takes off shoes and socks") is easier for girls by about 0.86 logits (= the difference in ability at the intersection of 50 per cent). Conversely, milestone ddigmm064 ("Crawls forward, abdomen on the floor") is easier for boys by about 0.84 logits. These are the most substantial differences found for sex in the DDI. Both are uniform DIF.

In practice, having milestones with opposite directions of DIF in the same instrument will cancel out one another, so one need not be overly concerned in

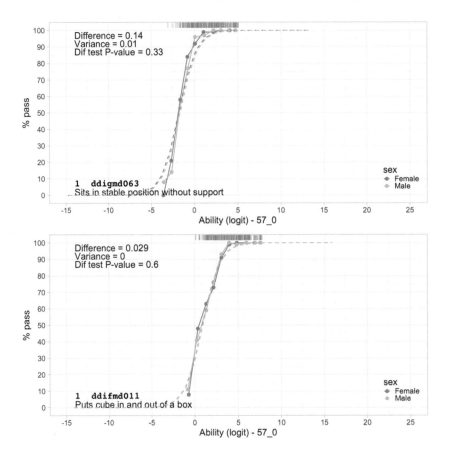

FIGURE 1.6.6 Two milestones from the DDI with similar item response curves for boys and girls. There is no DIF for sex.

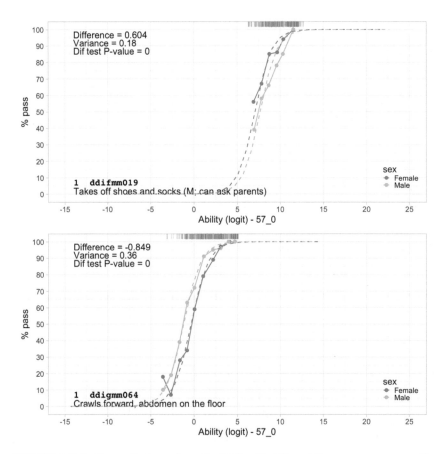

FIGURE 1.6.7 Two milestones from the DDI with different item response curves for boys and girls. There is evidence for uniform DIF.

that case. However, we should be careful when the tool consists of milestones that all have DIF in the same direction.

The DDI did not contain items for which the ability-group interaction was statistically significant, so we conclude that there is no non-uniform DIF in the DDI.

1.6.4 ITEM INFORMATION

1.6.4.1 ITEM INFORMATION AT A GIVEN ABILITY

Items are generally sensitive to only a part of the ability scale. Item information is a psychometric measure that quantifies how illuminating the item is at different levels of ability. We may visualize item information as a curve per item.

The formula to obtain the item information is the first derivative of the item response curve and can be written as follows:

$$I(\hat{\delta}_i) = P(\hat{\delta}_i)(1 - P(\hat{\delta}_i))$$

where $P(\hat{\delta}_i)$ is the conditional probability of endorsing item i, and where $\hat{\delta}_i$ is the estimated item difficulty in the logit scale. For example for milestone `ddicmm039` ("Says three words") $\hat{\delta}_i$ equals 4.06.

Figure 1.6.8 displays the item information curves for two milestones from the DDI. Note that the amount of information for the item is maximal around the item difficulty.

The probability of endorsing milestone `ddicmm039` for a child with an ability of 2 logits is

$$P_{ni} = \frac{\exp(2 - 4.06)}{1 + \exp(2 - 4.06)} = 0.113$$

At this ability level, milestone `ddicmm039` has information

$$I(\hat{\delta}_i) = 0.113 \times (1 - 0.113) = 0.10$$

1.6.4.2   ITEM INFORMATION AT A GIVEN AGE

In practice, it is often interesting to express the item information against age. By doing so, one can identify at what ages an item provides the most information.

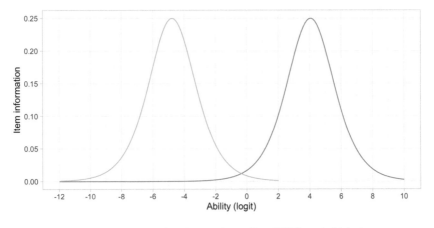

— ddicmm039 Says three 'words'   — ddigmm060 Rolls over back to front

FIGURE 1.6.8   The item information curve for two milestones from the DDI.

Figure 1.6.9 shows that the sensitive age ranges differ considerably between items. Suppose we use 0.05 as a criterion. Then `ddigmm060` is susceptible between ages 4–8 months, a period of four months. Item `ddicmm039` is receptive in the period 10–19 months, a range that is about twice as broad. The symmetric nature of the curves in Figure 1.6.8 is not present in Figure 1.6.9. In general, the relation between age and item sensitivity is more complicated than the relationship between ability and item sensitivity.

The item information by age curve helps to determine at what ages we should administer the item. The item will be most informative if delivered at the age at which 50% of the children will pass the milestone. This age corresponds to an item information is equal to 0.5 x 0.5 = 0.25. Administering the item closely around that age provide the most efficient measurement of ability. When space is at a premium (e.g. as in population surveys) using a well-chosen set of age-sensitive milestones will help in reducing the total number of milestones.

In other contexts, milestones may be used as a screening instrument to identify developmental delay. In that case, it is more efficient to administer items that are very easy for the age, e.g. milestones on which, say, 90% of the children will pass.

1.6.5 RELIABILITY

The reliability is a one-number summary of the accuracy of an instrument. Statisticians define reliability as the proportion of variance attributable to the variation between children's abilities relative to the total variance. More specifically, the reliability R of a test is written as

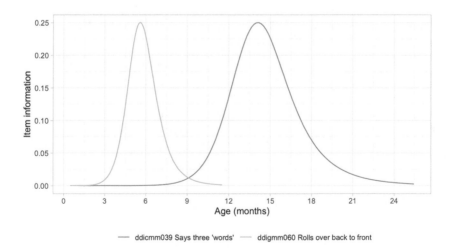

FIGURE 1.6.9 Information information of Figure 1.6.8 plotted against age.

$$R \equiv \frac{\sigma_\beta^2}{\sigma_\beta^2 + \sigma_e^2},$$

where σ_β^2 is the variance of true scores and σ_e^2 is the error variance.

In general, high reliability is desirable. We often use reliability to decide between instruments. Cronbach's α is a widely used estimate of the lower bound of the reliability of a test. In the Rasch model, we can estimate reliability by the ratio

$$\widehat{R} = \frac{\widehat{\sigma}_{\widehat{\beta}}^2 - \widehat{\sigma}_{\widehat{e}}^2}{\widehat{\sigma}_{\widehat{\beta}}^2}.$$

For a given model, we can calculate $\widehat{\sigma}_{\widehat{\beta}}^2$ directly as the sampling variance of the estimated abilities. Getting an estimate for $\widehat{\sigma}_{\widehat{e}}^2$ is more complicated. We use the modelled person abilities and item difficulties to generate a hypothetical data set of the same size and same missing data pattern, and re-estimate the person ability from the simulated data. Then $\widehat{\sigma}_{\widehat{e}}^2$ is computable as the variance of the difference between the modelled and re-estimated person ability.

The estimated variance of the modelled abilities is $\widehat{\sigma}_{\widehat{\beta}}^2 = 76.6$, and the variance of the difference between modelled and re-estimated abilities is equal to $\widehat{\sigma}_{\widehat{e}}^2 = 1.74$. The corresponding *standard error of measurement (sem)* is $\widehat{\sigma}_{\widehat{e}} = 1.32$ logits.

The estimated reliability in the SMOCC data is equal to $(76.6 - 1.74)/76.6 = 0.977$. We may interpret this estimate in the same way as Cronbach's α, for which typically any value beyond 0.9 is classified as *excellent*. Note that the reliability is very high because of the large variation in D-scores. Newborns are very different from 2-year old toddlers, which helps to increase reliability. In practice, it is perhaps more useful to use a measure of accuracy that is less dependent on the variation within the sample. The *sem*, as explained above, seems to be a more relevant measure of precision.

1.7 Validity

Stef van Buuren[1,2]
Iris Eekhout[1]
[1]Netherlands Organisation for Applied Scientific
Research TNO, Leiden, 2316 ZL, The Netherlands
[2]University of Utrecht, Utrecht, 3584 CH, The
Netherlands

Validity is a generic term that refers to the question of how well an instrument measures what it claims to measure. There are various aspects of validity. This section briefly reviews the main types of validity:

- Internal validity (1.7.1)
- External validity (1.7.2)

1.7.1 INTERNAL VALIDITY

1.7.1.1 CONTENT VALIDITY

Content validity is the extent to which the D-score represents all facets of development. In contrast to "face validity," which assesses whether the test appears valid to respondents, content validity is about what is measured.

One important form of content validity is that we wish to make sure that the measurement scale represents the various developmental domains in a fair way. In the simplest case, we can assign each milestone uniquely to one domain and evaluate coverage by splitting the cumulative item information.

Figure 1.7.1 shows the coverage of the three domains of the DDI at various levels of the D-score. The three domains of the DDI are relevant at most ability

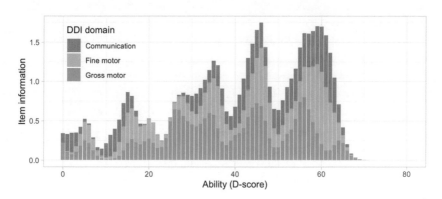

FIGURE 1.7.1 Cumulative item information by DDI domain.

DOI: 10.1201/9781003216315-7

levels. The DDI contains no communication milestones between 20 D and 30 D, so at these levels, the DDI measures primarily motor performance.

Content validity assessment is part of modelling when we examine what milestones fit the model. Content validity also means that all relevant facets of development are measured. As discussed in Section 1.6.1, we may remove items that do not fit the model and hence fail to measure development in the technical sense. As a result, we may lose items considered relevant by subject-matter specialists. If we want to preserve these, we could fit a separate model that captures another development aspect. We did not encounter the issue with the DDI. In contrast, our finding that items allocated to different domains form a unidimensional scale underlines the content validity of the D-score.

1.7.1.2 CONSTRUCT VALIDITY

Construct validity is the extent to which the D-score behaves like the theory says the construct should behave. For example, we expect that child development advances with age. Figure 1.4.3 provides convincing evidence that the D-score increases fastest in the first six months and keeps rising at a slower rate as children age. This phenomenon is consistent with theories in growth and child development.

In Section 1.4, we assumed that child development is a latent variable. Figure 1.7.2 provides one way to evaluate the validity of this assumption. The figure plots the item fit for each milestone coloured by domain. Items from different domains fit equally well, so there is no evidence that the D-score favours a particular area. Put in more technical terms; the DDI domains do not explain differences in the item fit residuals of the model.

1.7.2 EXTERNAL VALIDITY

1.7.2.1 DISCRIMINATORY VALIDITY

Discriminatory validity indicates the extent to which the D-score can distinguish children with non-normal development from children that are developing normally. We may evaluate this by identifying children with lagging development, for example, indicated by reflex or tonus problems, and study whether the D-score can discriminate those children from the general population. Section 1.9.3 presents some examples.

1.7.2.2 CONVERGENT AND DIVERGENT VALIDITY

Convergent validity is the extent to which the D-score relates to similar constructs. We measure it by the correlation between the D-score and the total score on Bayley-III or Denver.

The correlation with the other construct should be 0.6, or higher for good convergent validity. Unfortunately, at present, only limited data is available for the DDI, so we cannot assess convergent validity for the D-score at this point.

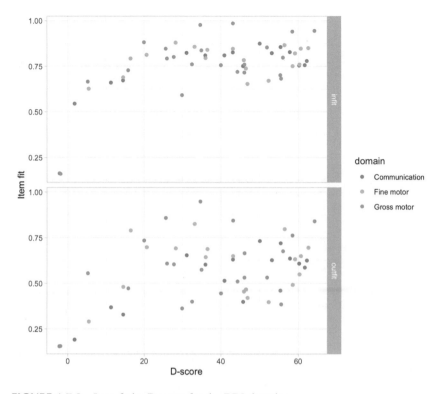

FIGURE 1.7.2   Item fit by D-score for the DDI domains.

Divergent validity is the extent to the D-score is uncorrelated with measures of a different construct.

Figure 1.7.3 shows both convergent and divergent validity at work. The figure shows that, as expected, there is a strong and almost linear relation between body height and the D-score. However, after correction for the child's age, the relationship between height and D-score almost disappears. Thus, growth and development are entirely different concepts.

We can also evaluate the strength of the relations between the D-score and proxy measures of child development, such as stunted height growth (see section 1.1.3). The low correlation between DAZ and HAZ suggests that stunting is a poor proxy for child development.

1.7.2.3   PREDICTIVE VALIDITY

Predictive validity refers to the degree to which the D-score predicts the score on a criterion that is measured later. For the D-score, we may compare to measures for IQ at the school-age as a possible criterion.

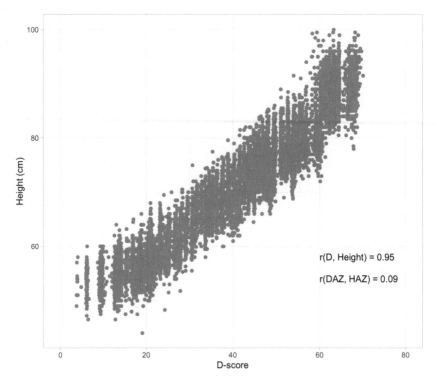

FIGURE 1.7.3   Relation between body height and the D-score in the SMOCC data.

Vlasblom *et al.* (2019) found strong evidence that individual milestones of the DDI measured during the first years of life predict later intellectual functioning at ages 5–10 years. It is to be expected that the D-score, which builds upon these individual items, will also predict limited intellectual functioning, perhaps even better.

1.8 Precision

Stef van Buuren[1,2]
Iris Eekhout[1]
with Manon Grevinga
[1]Netherlands Organisation for Applied Scientific Research TNO, Leiden, 2316 ZL, The Netherlands
[2]University of Utrecht, Utrecht, 3584 CH, The Netherlands

This section shows the properties of the D-score when calculated from short tests. The study of quick tests is useful because it reveals the behaviour of the D-score when the measurement is inherently imprecise.

This section covers:

- Structure of milestone subsets (1.8.1)
- Impact of short tests on D-score (1.8.2)
- Impact of short tests on predicting IQ (1.8.3)

1.8.1 SMOCC DESIGN: STANDARD AND ADDITIONAL MILESTONES

At each visit, the SMOCC study collected scores on a set of *standard milestones* (that about 90 per cent of the children will pass) and a set of *additional milestones* (that about 50 per cent of the children will pass). See Section 1.4.1.2.

The SMOCC dataset covers nine different *waves*. The set of milestones used in the DDI varies per visit. The number of standard milestones varies between 2

TABLE 1.8.1
Number of items administered per wave in the SMOCC data.

Age	Standard	Additional
1m	5	2
2m	2	5
3m	5	6
6m	6	7
9m	7	6
12m	6	6
15m	6	6
18m	6	7
24m	7	7

DOI: 10.1201/9781003216315-8

and 7 on various occasions. The additional milestones equal the standard ones from the next wave.

Table 1.8.1 summarizes the scheduled age for each wave, the number of standard milestones and the number of additional milestones.

Figure 1.8.1 shows the subsets of DDI items administered at each age. For example, at the 1-month visit, the five standard milestones are `ddicmm029 - ddigm056`, and the two additional ones are `ddicmm030` and `ddifmd002`. At the 2-month visit, the standard milestones are `ddicmm030` and `ddifmd002`, and the five additional ones are `ddicmm031 - ddigmd057`. And so on.

1.8.2   D-SCORE FROM SHORT TESTS

1.8.2.1   Milestone sets

In the analyses done thus far, we have calculated D-scores from responses on the combined (standard plus additional) milestones. Thus, at the 2-month visit, the D-score was calculated from 2 (standard) + 5 (additional) = 7 milestones.

In daily practice, the set of additional milestones is often lacking. This section explores the impact of using the (smaller) subset of standard milestones on measurement error and prediction.

This section reports and compares three D-scores:

1. D-score from standard milestones;
2. D-score from additional milestones.
3. D-score from all available milestones;

Estimation of 1 is more complicated than for 2 and 3, for the following reasons:

- There are fewer milestones, so the estimate is less precise and more influenced by choice of the prior distribution;
- The standard set contains only easy milestones, which are uninformative for the majority of children.

1.8.2.2   Milestone sets at month 2

The vertical axis of Figure 1.8.2 shows the D-score, separately calculated from the standard, additional and all milestones for children aged two months. The colour of the dots represents the number of FAIL ratings within each set of milestones.

At month two there are just two standard milestones: `ddicmm030` and `ddifmd002`. About 90 per cent of the infants will pass these. The green dots in the left-hand panel represent the estimated D-scores corresponding to two passes. As explained in Section 1.5.3.2, we calculate the D-score with an age-dependent prior. If the ages vary (and they do), then the D-score for infants having the same total score will also vary.

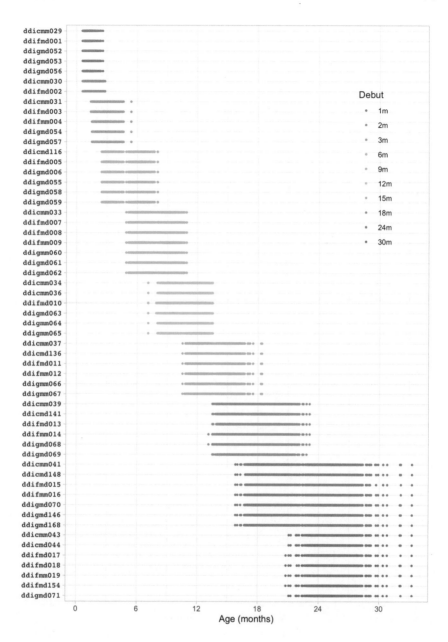

FIGURE 1.8.1 Age-item grid of the SMOCC study, illustrating how the 57 DDI items are distributed over nine visits during the first 24 months.

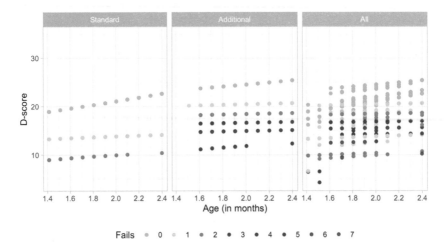

FIGURE 1.8.2 Distribution of the D-scores calculated from the standard, additional and all available milestones at month 2. Colors correspond to the number of fails.

If a child fails either `ddicmm030` or `ddifmd002`, then the D-score is substantially lower. The left-hand figure shows a *gap* between the green dots (perfect score) and the yellow dots (one FAIL). The impact of a FAIL on the D-score is substantial. For example, the D-score of an infant with one FAIL on a standard milestone drops from about 20 D to 14 D. Thus, with these two milestones, there cannot be a D-score in the range 15 D - 18 D. It depends on the purposes of the measurement if this is acceptable. We can prevent gaps by measuring more milestones, e.g., milestones taken from the additional set. Another gap occurs between 14 D and 11 D. These gaps illustrate that precision is constrained if we administer only two milestones.

The middle panel shows the estimated D-score at the same visit but now calculated from the five additional milestones (i.e., the standard milestones from month 3). Infant aged two months have approximately a 50 per cent chance of passing each. Note that administration of the additional milestones will cover the range 14D-20 D quite well. Note the ceiling is also higher with these milestones.

Note that the range of the estimated D-scores is quite similar in both plots. This similarity is a result of accounting for the difficulty level of milestones. The estimate of the D-score is *unbiased* for difficulty.

The panel on the right-hand side provides the D-score calculated from all milestones. We can easily recognize the points coming from the standard and additional sets. Also, there is a limited number of ratings on easier items that belong to month 1. We rescored these because the child failed these milestones at the previous visit. Rescoring effectively extends the range of possible D-scores to the lower end, so now we can find some children who have D-score lower than 10 D.

1.8.2.3   MILESTONE SETS AT MONTH 3

Figure 1.8.3 is the same plot as before, but now for month 3. Compared to Figure 1.8.2, all points shifted upwards because the children are now one month older.

The additional milestones from month 2 are the standard milestones of month 3. In Figure 1.8.2, there were at least 11 children (in purple) failed all five additional milestones. One month later, one child has five fails.

1.8.2.4   FLOOR AND CEILING EFFECTS

Figure 1.8.4 plot the D-score distribution for all occasions. Some observations:

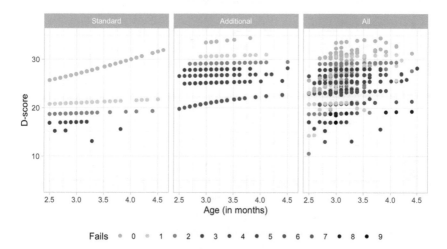

FIGURE 1.8.3   Distribution of the D-scores calculated from the standard, additional and all available milestones at month 3. Colors correspond to the number of fails.

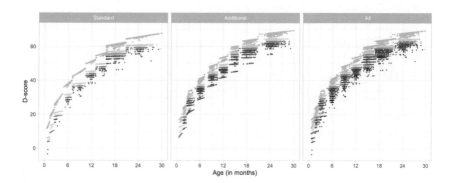

FIGURE 1.8.4   D-score by age 0–30 months for standard, additional and all available milestones at each measurement occasion.

- *Ceiling effect*: The ceiling effect (green) is most prominent in the *standard* set, but is also present in the other two sets. None of the three sets can filter out children with really advanced development. To achieve more precision at the upper end, we would need to include more difficult milestones.
- *Floor effect*: There are almost no floor effects in the *standard* and *all* sets. These sets discriminate well among children with delayed development, which was the designed purpose of the DDI. Note that floor effects are visible in the *additional* set.
- *Average level*: All three sets capture the overall relation between age and development. The *additional* set is quite efficient for measuring average levels development but lacks detail on the extremes.

Figure 1.8.4 shows that a short test (5–6 milestones) can precisely measure the lower tail of the D-score distribution (*standard* set) or the middle of the D-score distribution (*additional* set), but cannot do both at the same time.

1.8.3   IMPACT OF SHORT TESTS ON PREDICTING IQ

1.8.3.1   MEASUREMENT AND PREDICTION

In Section 1.8.2, we saw that a short test can measure the middle or one tail of the distribution, but cannot be precise for both at the same time. If we want to identify children at risk for delayed development, we are interested in the lower tail of the distribution, so in that case, the *standard* set is suitable. But what set should we use if we want to predict a later outcome?

This section explores that effect of taking different milestone sets on the quality of prediction.

1.8.3.2   UKKI

Hafkamp-de Groen *et al.* (2009) studied the effect of the D-score on later intelligence, using a subset of 557 SMOCC children that were followed up at the age of five years.

The Utrechtse Korte Kleuter Intelligentietest (UKKI) (Baarda, 1978) is a short test to measure intelligence. The UKKI is a simple test with just three components:

- Redraw five figures (square, triangle, cross, trapezoid, rhomboid);
- Draw human figure, with 28 characteristics, like legs, eyes, and so on;
- Give meaning to 13 words like knife, banana, umbrella, and so on.

Administration time is about 15–20 minutes. The UKKI has a reasonable test-retest reliability for group use (Pearson $r = 0.74$, 3-month interval).

1.8.3.3 EXPLORATORY ANALYSIS

Figure 1.8.5 shows the empirical IQ distribution of 557 children. The mean IQ score is 108, and the standard deviation is 15, so the IQ scores of children in the sample is about a half standard deviation above the 1978 reference sample.

Figure 1.8.6 shows that the relation between the D-score 0–2 years and IQ at five years is positive for all milestone sets and all ages. The strength of the association increases with age. At the age of 2 years, the regression coefficient for D-score is equal to β (D) = 1.4 (SE: 0.21, p < 0.0001), so on average an

---

TABLE 1.8.2

Pearson correlation between D-score (0–2 years) and IQ at 5 years.

Visit	Standard set	Additional set	All milestones
1m	0.059	0.005	0.027
2m	0.051	0.056	0.048
3m	0.036	0.100	0.102
6m	0.040	0.038	0.036
9m	0.094	0.143	0.132
12m	0.046	0.162	0.137
15m	0.180	0.153	0.187
18m	0.129	0.153	0.146
24m	0.245	0.255	0.267

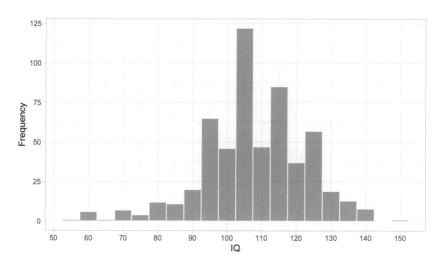

FIGURE 1.8.5 Histogram of UKKI *IQ* scores taken around the age of five years (SMOCC data, n = 557).

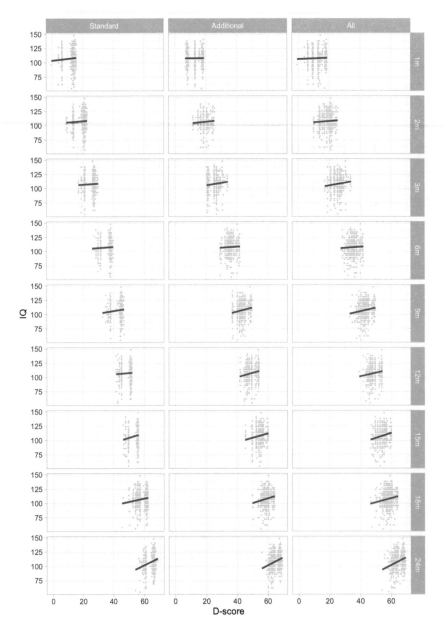

FIGURE 1.8.6   Relation between D-score at infancy and *IQ* at age 5 years according to three milestone sets and nine visits (SMOCC data, *n* = 557).

increase of 1.0 unit in the D-score at the age of 2 years corresponds to a 1.4 IQ-score points increase at the age five years.

Table 1.8.2 summarizes the Pearson correlations between the D-score and later IQ. The association between D-score and IQ is weak during the first year of life but gets stronger during the second year. In general, having more (and more informative) milestones helps to increase the correlation, but the effects are relatively small. So even from the standard set of the seven easy milestones at 24m, we obtain a reasonable correlation of 0.245.

All in all, these results suggest that neither the amount nor the difficulty level of the milestones is critical in determining the strength of the relation between the D-score and IQ.

1.9 Three studies

Stef van Buuren[1,2]
Iris Eekhout[1]
with Paula van Dommelen
Maria C. Olthof
[1]Netherlands Organisation for Applied Scientific
Research TNO, Leiden, 2316 ZL, The Netherlands
[2]University of Utrecht, Utrecht, 3584 CH, The
Netherlands

This section compares child development between samples from three different studies:

- *SMOCC*, a representative sample of Dutch children (1.9.1)
- *POPS*, a cohort of all Dutch preterms in 1983 (1.9.2)
- *TOGO*, a set of medical records from preventive health service in Togo (1.9.3)
- A summary of the main findings (1.9.4)

Each study used the same measurement instrument, the DDI (see Section 1.4.1). The section compares D-scores between studies.

1.9.1 SMOCC STUDY

Figure 1.9.1 shows the D-score distribution by age in the SMOCC data. The grey curves represent references calculated from the SMOCC data. The top figure illustrates that rise of the D-score with age, whereas the bottom chart shows that the DAZ distribution covers the references well.

The ceiling effect causes low coverage after the age of 24 months. There are also less prominent ceiling effects for younger children. Without these effects, the references would presumably show some additional variation.

1.9.2 POPS STUDY

Figure 1.9.2 presents the D-score and DAZ distributions for the POPS cohort of children born very preterm or with very low birth weight. The distributions of the D-score and DAZ are similar to those found in the SMOCC study.

Since the D-scores are calculated using the same milestones and difficulty estimates as used in the SMOCC data, the D-scores are comparable across the two studies. When the milestones differ between studies (e.g. when studies use

DOI: 10.1201/9781003216315-9

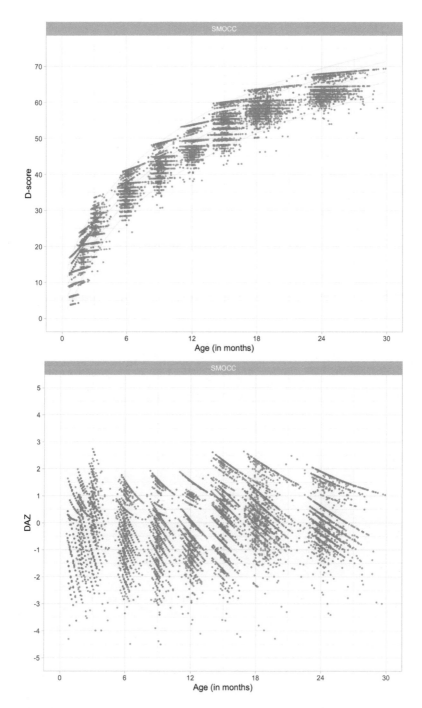

FIGURE 1.9.1   Distribution of D-score and DAZ by child age in a cohort of Dutch children aged 0–2 years (Source: SMOCC data, *n* = 2151, 9 occasions).

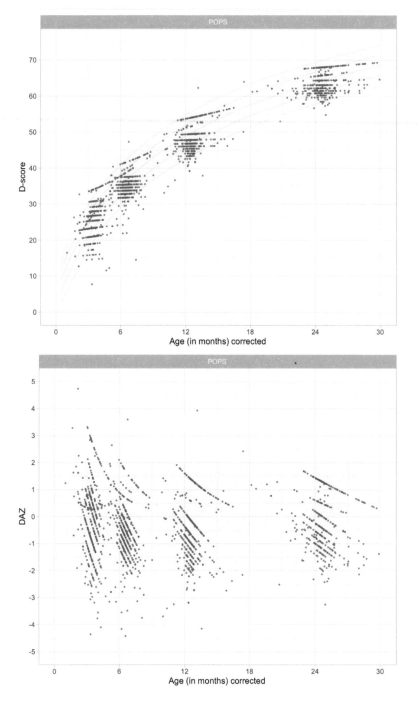

FIGURE 1.9.2   Distribution of D-score and DAZ by child age in a cohort of preterm aged 0–2 years.

different measurement instruments), it is still possible to calculate D-scores. This problem is a little more complicated, so we treat it in Chapter 2.

The primary new complication here is the question whether it is fair to compare *postnatal age* of children born at term with postnatal ages of very preterm children. This section focuses on this issue in some detail.

1.9.2.1 POPS DESIGN

In 1983, the Project On Preterm and Small for Gestational Age Infants (POPS study) collected data on all 1338 infants in the Netherlands who had very preterm birth (gestational age < 32 weeks) or very low birth weight (birth weight < 1500 grams). See Verloove - Vanhorick *et al.* (1986) for details.

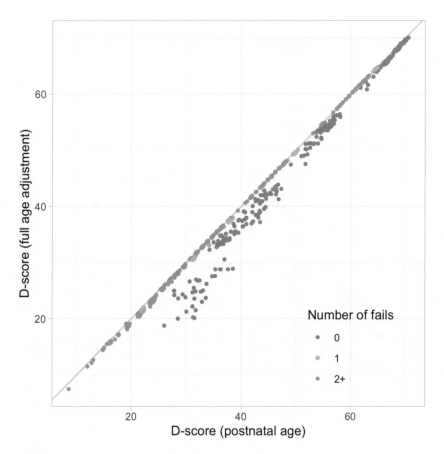

FIGURE 1.9.3 Scatterplot of two versions of the D-score, one calculated using postnatal age ($f = 0.00$), the other calculated using full age-adjustment ($f = 1.00$).

The POPS study determined gestational age from the best obstetric estimate, including the last menstrual period, results of pregnancy testing, and ultrasonography findings. The POPS study collected measurements on 450 children using the DDI at four visits at corrected postnatal ages of 3, 6, 12 and 24 months.

1.9.2.2 AGE-ADJUSTMENT

Assessment of very preterm children at the same chronological age as term children may cause over-diagnosis of developmental delay in very preterm children. Very preterm children may require additional time that allows for development equivalent to that of children born a term.

In anthropometry, it is common to correct chronological age of very preterm born children to enable age-appropriate evaluation of growth. For example, suppose the child is born as a gestational age of 30 weeks, which is ten weeks early. A *full correction* would deduct ten weeks from the child's postnatal age, and a *half correction* would deduct five weeks. In particular, we calculate the corrected age (in days) as:

$$\text{corrected age} = \text{postnatal age (days)} - f \times [280 - \text{gestational age (days)}],$$

where 280 is the average gestational age in days, and where we specify several alternatives for f as 1.00 (full correction), 0.75, 0.50 (half) or 0.00 (no correction).

Let's apply the same idea to child development. Using *corrected age* instead of *postnatal age* has two consequences:

- It will affect the prior distribution for calculating the D-score;
- It will affect DAZ calculation.

We evaluate these two effects in turn.

1.9.2.3 EFFECT OF AGE-ADJUSTMENT ON THE D-SCORE

Figure 1.9.3 plots the fully age-adjusted D-score against the unadjusted D-score. Any discrepancies result only from differences in the ages used in the age-dependent prior (cf. Section 1.5.3.2).

All points are on or below the diagonal. Age-adjustment lowers the D-score because a preterm is "made younger" by subtracting the missed pregnancy duration, and hence the prior distribution starts at the lower point. For example, the group of red marks with D-scores between 30 D and 40 D (age not corrected) will have D-scores between 20 D and 30 D when fully corrected. Note that only the red points (with perfect scores) are affected, thus illustrating that the prior has its most significant effect on the perfect response pattern. See also Section 1.5.3.1. The impact of age-correction on the D-score is negligible when the child fails on one or more milestones.

1.9.2.4 EFFECT OF NO AGE ADJUSTMENT ($F = 0.00$) ON THE DAZ

Figure 1.9.4 illustrates that a considerable number of D-scores fall below the minus -2 SD line of the reference when age is not adjusted, especially during the first year of life. The pattern suggests that the apparent slowness in development is primarily the result of being born early, and does not necessarily reflect delayed development.

1.9.2.5 EFFECT OF FULL AGE ADJUSTMENT ($F = 0.00$) ON THE DAZ

Full age correction has a notable effect on the DAZ. Figure 1.9.5 illustrates that the POPS children are now somewhat advanced over the reference children. We ascribe this seemingly odd finding to more prolonged exposure to sound and vision in air. Thus after age correction, development in preterms during early infancy is advanced compared to just-born babies.

Full age correction seems to overcorrect the D-score, so it is natural to try intermediate values for f between 0 and 1.

1.9.2.6 PARTIAL AGE ADJUSTMENT

Table 1.9.1 compares mean DAZ under various specifications for f. Values $f = 0.00$ and $f = 0.50$ do not correct for preterm birth enough in the sense that all sign are negative. In contrast, $f = 1.00$ overcorrects. The value of 0.73 is implausibly high, especially because this value is close to birth. Setting $f = 0.75$ seems a good compromise, in the sense that the average DAZ is close to zero in the first age interval. The average DAZ is negative at later ages. We do not know whether this genuinely reflects less than optimal development of very preterm and low birth weight children, so either $f = 1.00$ and $f = 0.75$ are suitable candidates.

TABLE 1.9.1
Average DAZ at various ages under four correction factors.

Age (months)	0.00	0.50	0.75	1.00
0–3	-1.46	-0.50	0.07	0.73
3–4	-1.77	-0.89	-0.37	0.20
5–6	-1.60	-0.87	-0.46	0.00
7–8	-1.76	-1.13	-0.77	-0.39
9—1	-1.21	-0.77	-0.53	-0.28
12–14	-0.99	-0.60	-0.39	-0.16
15–23	-0.50	-0.23	-0.10	0.04
24+	-0.70	-0.49	-0.37	-0.24

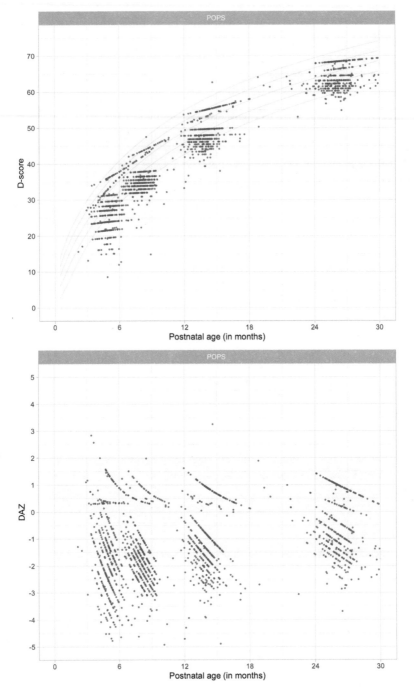

FIGURE 1.9.4   Distribution of D-score and DAZ without age correction for preterm birth ($f = 0.00$).

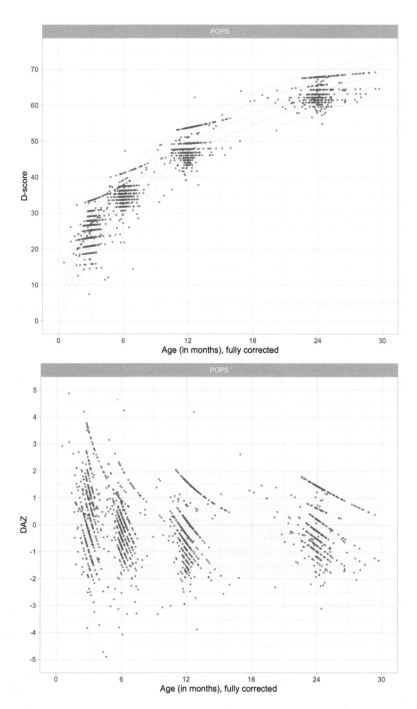

FIGURE 1.9.5   Distribution of D-score and DAZ under full age correction for preterm birth ($f = 1.00$).

1.9.2.7 CONCLUSIONS

- Compared with the general population, more very preterm children reached developmental milestones within chronological age five months when chronological age was fully corrected;
- Fewer preterm children reached the milestones when chronological age was not corrected;
- Fewer children reached the milestones when we used a correction of $f = 0.50$;
- Similar proportions were observed when we used $f = 0.75$ within the first five months after birth.
- After chronological age five months, we observed similar proportions for very preterm and full-term children when chronological age was fully corrected.
- We recommend using full age correction ($f = 1.00$). This advice corresponds to current practice for growth and development. As we have shown, preterms may look better in the first few months under full age-correction. If the focus of the scientific study is on the first few months, we recommend an age correction of $f = 0.75$.

1.9.3 TOGO STUDY

Figure 1.9.6 presents the D-score and DAZ distributions of a sample of children living near Kpalimé, Togo. While the primary trend with age conforms to the previous data, the distributions differ from those in Figure 1.9.1 and Figure 1.9.2 in two respects:

- *Compression at the upper end*: Most of the D-scores are above the median curve, which suggests that, at these ages, children living in Togo *develop faster* than children living in the Netherlands;
- *Expansion at the lower end*: There is a considerable variation in D-scores on the lower end, with many D-scores below the -2 SD curve, suggesting that some children are *significantly more delayed* than would be expected in both Dutch samples.

The D-scores are calculated using the same 57 milestones and difficulty estimates as before. The resulting D-score distribution is quite unusual. The main question here is what could explain the pattern found in the D-scores. This section explores this question in some detail.

1.9.3.1 TOGO KPALIMÉ STUDY, DESIGN

If the D-score is to be a universal measure, then it should be informative in *low and middle-income countries* (LMIC) as well. We do not yet know much about the usability and validity of the D-score in LMIC's. The western African country of Togo qualifies as a low-income country, with a 2017 GNI per

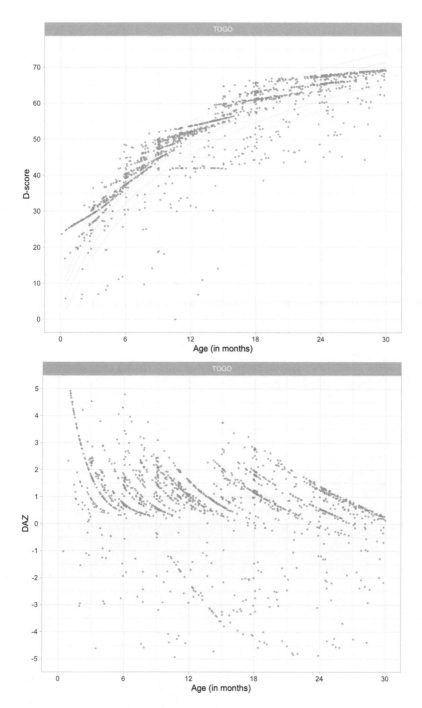

FIGURE 1.9.6 Distribution of D-score and DAZ by child age of children living near Kpalimé, Togo (Source: TOGO data),

capita of USD 610, compared to USD 46,180 in the Netherlands, and USD 744 for low-income countries in general (data.worldbank.org).

The data were collected by Cécile Schat-Savy, who initiated a youth health care centre modelled after the Dutch youth health care system in Kpalimé, Togo. See https://www.kinderhulp-togo.nl for more background. Data monitoring included a french translation the DDI for measuring child development. The investigators gathered data from 9747 individuals in the 0–18 age range.

Participants include children and their parents who visited the Kpalimé health centre at least one time. Kpalimé is the fourth largest town in Togo, but the health centre also attracted parents and children from a wide surrounding rural area. Parents visited the health centre for several reasons, including for a preventive health check or because of their child's apparent health problems.

The health centre targeted parents through information sessions for parents at primary schools. Parents paid a small amount of money per child (about USD 4.00 for children of 4 years or older, and USD 0.80 for children younger than four years). Four local data-assistants, some portrayed in Figure 1.9.7, digitized the data from paper archives. TNO Child Health in The Netherlands monitored the process and checked the data for completeness and consistency.

Here we use a subset of 2674 visits from 1644 unique children who scored on the 57 milestones of the DDI 0–2 years. We did not calculate D-scores when age or DDI milestones were missing, which left a dataset of 2425 visits from unique 1567 children. The number of visits varied from 1 – 9. The majority of children visited the centre once.

1.9.3.2 D-SCORE LABELLED BY NEUROLOGICAL PROBLEM

Figure 1.9.8 is the same scatter plot as in Figure 1.9.6, but now marked by whether the physician registered signs of neuropathology in the form of tonus and reflex problems.

Many children with low D-scores also have tonus or reflex problems. This finding alone suggests that extreme D-score are not artefacts (e.g. caused by a wrongly coded age), but indicate main adverse health conditions.

1.9.3.3 D-SCORE LABELLED BY APGAR SCORE

Figure 1.9.9 identifies the children who had an Apgar score at 10 minutes after birth that was lower than 8. About half of these children had a D-score below -2 SD curve.

1.9.3.4 D-SCORE LABELLED BY SEVERE UNDERWEIGHT

Many children who visited the Kpalimé health centre had a low body weight for their age. Figure 1.9.10 marks the subset of severely underweight children (WAZ < -4). A substantial proportion of these children also had a very low D-score.

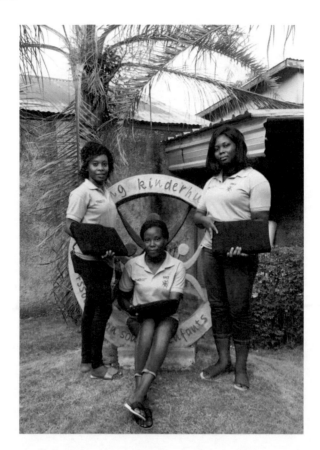

FIGURE 1.9.7   Three of the data-assistants who helped to digitize the paper files.

Reproduced with permission from Stichting Kinderhulp Togo https://www.kinderhulp-togo.nl.

1.9.3.5   D-SCORE LABELLED BY SEVERE STUNTING

Figure 1.9.11 is similar to 1.9.10, but now marked by the subset of severely stunted children (HAZ < -4). Also here, a sizable proportion has a low D-score.

When taken together, Figure 1.9.8–Figure 1.9.11 show that children with very low D-scores often experience (multiple) harsh health problems. Those health problems may have substantially delayed their development.

1.9.3.6   GROSS MOTOR DEVELOPMENT

Figure 1.9.12 shows substantial differences in gross motor development between children from Togo and the Netherlands. For example, at the age of three months, about 30 per cent of the Dutch infants succeed in controlling their head when pulled to sitting. However, infants from Togo seem already capable of head control when they are just one month old.

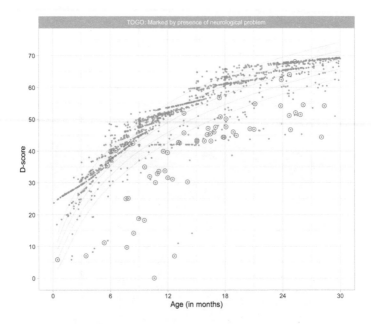

FIGURE 1.9.8   Distribution of D-score by age labelled by neurological (tonus and/or reflex) problems. (Source: TOGO data).

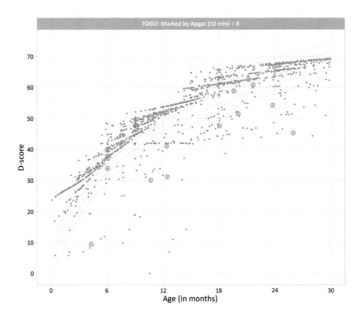

FIGURE 1.9.9   Distribution of D-score by age labelled by Apgar score (10 minutes) lower than 8.

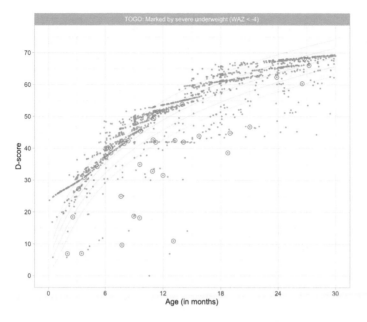

FIGURE 1.9.10   Distribution of D-score by age labelled by severe underweight (WAZ -4) (Source: TOGO data).

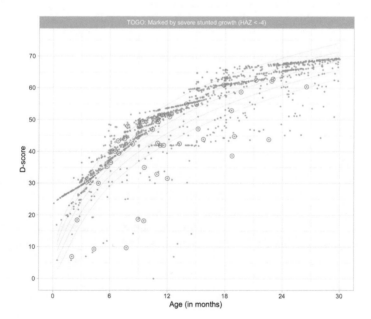

FIGURE 1.9.11   Distribution of D-score by age labelled by severe stunting (HAZ -4) (Source: TOGO data).

Moreover, the advantage persists at least until up to the age of two years: children in Togo can roll over and sit much earlier, or kick a ball without falling. As the documentary Babies shows, African children even manage to learn to walk with a tin can on their head, a craft that children in the west never achieve.

1.9.3.7 FINE MOTOR DEVELOPMENT

Figure 1.9.13 shows a less pronounced but similar phenomenon for fine motor skills. These data suggest that children in Togo may have better fine motor skills than the children from the two Dutch cohorts.

1.9.3.8 COMMUNICATION AND LANGUAGE

Figure 1.9.14 summarizes the data for three milestones on communication and language. In general, the success probability is similar in the three studies.

One curious finding is that the high proportion of milestones passes in ddicmm041 for the Togo children around the age of 18 months. Note that several of the green lines in Figure 1.9.12–Figure 1.9.14 start close to perfect scores, which makes it impossible to show the rising patterns found in the Dutch data.

It may indeed be true that children from Togo develop more rapidly than Dutch children. But we may also wonder: Could there just be reporting bias on the part of the parents who either do not understand the items or have the expectation to say "yes" even if the child can't do it? It would be desirable if these results could be backed up from other sources.

1.9.4 CONCLUSIONS

This section compared the D-scores estimated from the DDI administered to three different groups of children.

We found that

- The D-score by age plot showed a positive, curved relationship with age in all three studies;
- Children born very preterm or with very low birth weight had similar development to reference children when their age was corrected for early birth;
- A relatively small subset of children born in Togo had extremely low D-scores, not found in the Netherlands, likely the result of underlying neuropathology, severe underweight or severe stunting;
- On average, children from Togo seemed to have faster development during the first two years, especially in motor development, though there may be issues with reporting bias.

All in all, these findings support the usefulness and validity of the D-score as an informative summary of child development during their first two years of life.

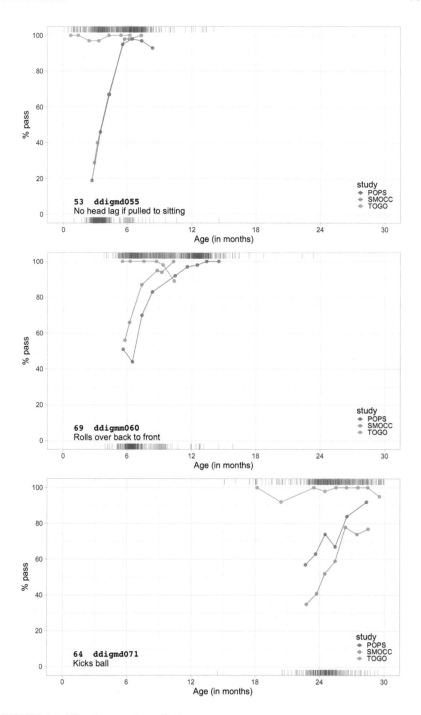

FIGURE 1.9.12 Gross motor milestones.

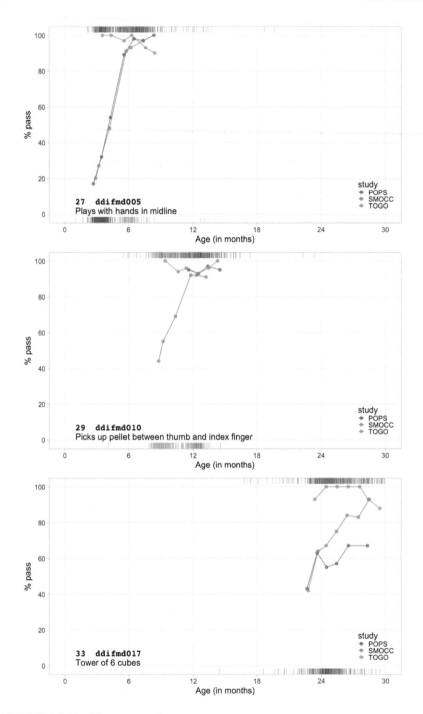

FIGURE 1.9.13   Fine motor milestones.

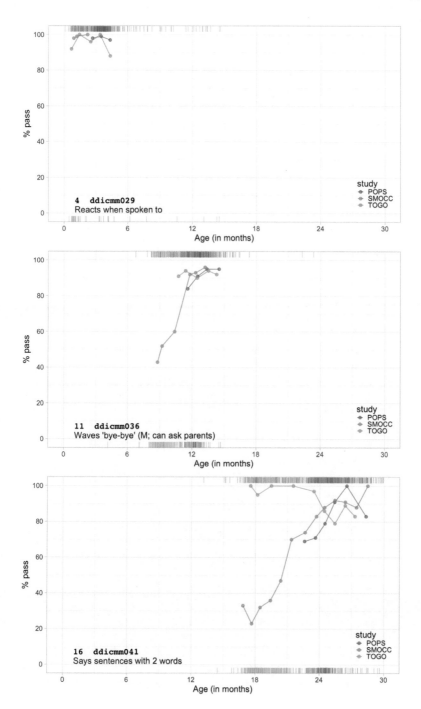

FIGURE 1.9.14   Communication and language milestones.

1.10 Next steps

Stef van Buuren[1,2]
Iris Eekhout[1]
[1]Netherlands Organisation for Applied
Scientific Research TNO, Leiden, 2316 ZL,
The Netherlands
[2]University of Utrecht, Utrecht, 3584 CH, The
Netherlands

This section provides a quick overview of the relevance, concepts and techniques of the D-score. While the results obtained thus far are encouraging, some questions will certainly remain when we put the method to practice.

A rough selection of such questions includes:

- What is the added value of the D-score in practice?
- Does the D-score extend to higher ages?
- Is the assumption of uni-dimensionality reasonable for other ages and populations?
- Can we calculate the D-score from instruments other than the DDI?
- Is it reasonable to assume that milestone difficulty is identical in other populations?
- Does the method apply to caregiver-reported milestones?
- Would a dedicated D-score instrument be more efficient?
- How many milestones are "enough"?
- Can the same scale be used for measurement at individual, group and population levels?
- Can the D-score detect delayed development?
- Would the D-score help to target early interventions?

This section briefly reviews some of these issues.

1.10.1 USEFULNESS OF D-SCORE FOR MONITORING CHILD HEALTH

The D-score is a new approach to measure child development. The D-score is a scale for quantifying generic child development by a single number. Milestones are selected to fit the Rasch model. We can interpret the resulting measurements as scores on an interval scale, a requirement for answering questions like:

- What is the difference in development over time for the same child, group or population?

DOI: 10.1201/9781003216315-10

- What is the difference in development between different children, groups or populations of the same age?
- How does child development compare to a norm?

The concept of the D-score is broader than a score calculated from the DDI. Any instrument that fits the model underlying the D-score can be used to measure the child's D-score.

The precision of the measurement depends on the number of milestones and the match between milestone difficulty and person ability. We may thus tailor the measurement instrument to the question at hand.

1.10.2   D-CHART, A GROWTH CHART FOR CHILD DEVELOPMENT

The field of child growth and development roughly divides into two areas:

- The subfield *child growth* (or *auxology*) emphasizes body measures like height, weight, body mass index, and so on. It is a rigorous quantitative science with intimate ties to statistics since the days of Quetelet and Galton.
- The subfield *child development* is more recent and builds upon a wide-ranging set of domain-specific instruments for measuring motor, language, cognitive and behavioural states.

The *growth chart* is a widely used tool to monitor physical growth. The D-score can be used in a similar way to create the *D-chart*.

Figure 1.10.1 shows the developmental paths of five randomly chosen children from the SMOCC study. Although the milestones differ across age, there is only one vertical axis. These trajectories will help to track the progress of a child over time.

The D-chart shows that it is straightforward to apply quantitative techniques from child growth to child development. Our hope is that D-score aids in bridging the disparate subfields of child growth and child development.

1.10.3   OPPORTUNITIES FOR EARLY INTERVENTION

Black *et al.* (2017) estimated that about 250 million children worldwide fail to reach their developmental potential. Developmental delays become evident in the first year and worsen during early childhood. The burden of children not reaching their developmental potential is high.

Interventions aimed at improving child development work best when delivered at the sensitive periods. Programs are to be comprehensive, incorporating a combination of health, nutrition, security and safety, responsive caregiving and early learning. See Engle *et al.* (2011); Grantham-McGregor *et al.* (2014) and Britto *et al.* (2017) for recent overviews and initiatives.

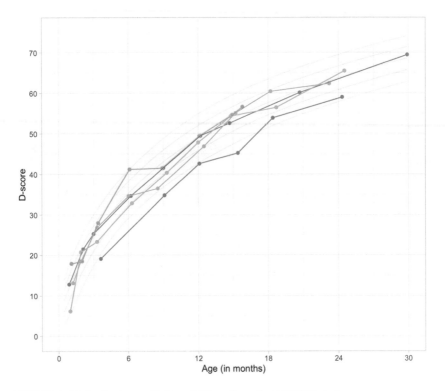

FIGURE 1.10.1 D-chart with five children from the SMOCC study.

The lack of a universal measure for child development has long hampered the ability to estimate intervention effects or to compare populations. The D-score can be generalized to other instruments. We expect that the availability of a common yardstick will stimulate informed policy and priority setting. We hope a universal measure improves decision making, ultimately lowering the number of children not reaching their developmental potential.

1.10.4 D-SCORE FOR INTERNATIONAL SETTINGS

Section 1.9 compared D-scores between three study samples. We restricted the analysis to studies that used the same instrument (the DDI, in Togo, translated to French) to measure child development.

It is difficult to compare levels of child development worldwide. Existing estimates on children not reaching their developmental potential rely on proxies, such as stunting and poverty. While these proxies have been found to correlate with child development, they are only weak indicators of actual child performance. Arguably, the performance of a child on a set of well-chosen milestones is more informative for his or her future health and productivity than body height or parental income.

There are more than 150 instruments are available that quantify child development. Many of these tools produce not just one but many scores. Such an overwhelming choice may seem a luxury until we realize that we cannot compare their ratings. Of course, we could settle on just one instrument ...., but that's never going to happen. While simple in theory, pre-harmonization is complicated in practice. It requires significant and continued investments by a central agency. It does not address historical data, so it will be challenging to see secular trends. Also, pre-harmonization impedes the adoption of innovative techniques, e.g., using smartphone-assisted evaluations.

The D-score opens up an exciting alternative: *agree on the scale*, and leave some liberty to the data-collector in the exact choice of the instrument. We could build upon the expertise of the data collector about the local population. Also, it will equip is to keep up with innovations in measurement.

The next chapter in our work will address some of the conceptual and technical issues that arise when we attempt to apply the D-score to other populations.

1.10.5   D-SCORE FROM EXISTING INSTRUMENTS

There is a vast base of historic child developmental data using existing instruments. The problem is that each device defines its own summaries, so we cannot compare scores across tools. Different instruments have different domains, various age forms, different stopping rules, diverse age norms, and so on. Yet, the milestones in these instruments are often very similar. Most tools collect data on milestones like:

- Can the child stack two blocks?
- Can the child roll over?
- Can the child draw a cross?
- Can the child stand?
- Can the child say "baba?"

With the D-score methodology in hand, we are ready to exploit the overlap in milestones shared by different instruments. Common items can act as *bridges*, so - with the appropriate item-level data - we may attempt calculating D-scores from other tools as well.

The task is to identify milestones that overlap between both instruments, filter out milestones that do not fit a joint model, and estimate the item difficulties of items that remain. Chapter 2 (van Buuren & Eekhout, 2021) will explore this possibility in more detail.

1.10.6   CREATING NEW INSTRUMENTS FOR D-SCORE

Extending the D-score to other instruments has the side-effect of enlarging the item bank with useful items. As more and more data feed into the item bank, assessment of already present milestones may become more precise.

The enlarged and improved item bank then may act as the fundamental resource for creating instruments for particular settings. For example, if the interest is on finding the most advanced children, we may construct a difficult test that will separate the good and the best. Alternatively, we can use the item bank to create and administer *computerized adaptive tests* (Jacobusse & van Buuren, 2007; Wainer *et al.*, 2000), a sequential method that selects the next milestone based on the previous test outcome.

Our ongoing work will explore the conceptual and technical challenges, and propose an integrated approach to support instrument construction and validation.

1.11 Appendices

Stef van Buuren[1,2]
Iris Eekhout[1]
[1]Netherlands Organisation for Applied Scientific Research TNO, Leiden, 2316 ZL, The Netherlands
[2]University of Utrecht, Utrecht, 3584 CH, The Netherlands

A - NOTATION

The notation in this chapter follows Wright & Masters (1982).

Section	Symbol	Term	Description
1.4.6	β_n	Ability	True (but unknown) developmental score of child n
1.4.6	δ_i	Difficulty	True (but unknown) difficulty of item i
1.4.6	π_{ni}	Probability	True (but unknown) probability that child n passes item i
1.6.1	$\hat{\beta}_n$	Ability	Estimated developmental score (D-score) of child n
1.6.1	$\hat{\delta}_i$	Difficulty	Estimated difficulty of item i
1.6.1	P_{ni}	Probability	Estimated probability that child n passes item i
1.6.1	x_{ni}	Data	Observed response of child n on item i, 0 or 1
1.6.1	W_{ni}	Variance	Variance of x_{ni}
1.6.1	z_{ni}	Residual	Standardized residual between x_{ni} and P_{ni}
1.6.1	N	Count	Number of measurements (children)
1.6.1	L	Count	Number of items (milestones)
1.6.4	$P(\hat{\delta}_i)$	Probability	Conditional probability of passing item i
1.6.4	$I(\hat{\delta}_i)$	Information	Item information function of item i
1.6.5	R	Reliability	True test reliability
1.6.5	$\hat{R}$	Reliability	Estimated test reliability
1.6.5	σ_e^2	Variance	True error variance
1.6.5	$\hat{\sigma}_{\hat{e}}^2$	Variance	Estimated error variance
1.6.5	$\hat{\sigma}_{\hat{e}}$	Variance	Standard error of measurement (sem)
1.9.2	f	Factor	Age-adjustment factor

B - TECHNICAL INFORMATION

```
R version 4.0.4 (2021-02-15)
Platform: x86_64-apple-darwin17.0 (64-bit)
Running under: macOS Big Sur 10.16
```

DOI: 10.1201/9781003216315-11

```
Matrix products: default
BLAS:      /Library/Frameworks/R.framework/Versions/4.0/Resources/lib/libRblas.
dylib
LAPACK:              /Library/Frameworks/R.framework/Versions/4.0/Resources/lib/
libRlapack.dylib

locale:
[1] en_US.UTF-8/en_US.UTF-8/en_US.UTF-8/C/en_US.UTF-8/en_US.UTF-8

attached base packages:
[1] stats     graphics  grDevices utils     datasets  methods   base

other attached packages:
 [1] dinstrument_0.0.1.2 ddata_0.52.0        gseddata_1.5.1
 [4] dmetric_0.52.0      dscore_1.4.0.9000   forcats_0.5.1
 [7] haven_2.3.1         scales_1.1.1        plotly_4.9.3
[10] sirt_3.9-4          gridExtra_2.3       plyr_1.8.6
[13] reshape2_1.4.4      RColorBrewer_1.1-2  dplyr_1.0.4
[16] tidyr_1.1.2         ggplot2_3.3.3       officer_0.3.17.001
[19] officedown_0.2.1    kableExtra_1.3.2    knitr_1.31

loaded via a namespace (and not attached):
 [1] nlme_3.1-152       webshot_0.5.2      httr_1.4.2        tools_4.0.4
 [5] R6_2.5.0           DBI_1.1.1          lazyeval_0.2.2    colorspace_2.0-0
 [9] withr_2.4.1        tidyselect_1.1.0  compiler_4.0.4    polycor_0.7-10
[13] rvest_0.3.6        TAM_3.5-19         xml2_1.3.2        bookdown_0.21
[17] mvtnorm_1.1-1      gamlss_5.2-0       systemfonts_1.0.1 stringr_1.4.0
[21] digest_0.6.27      rmarkdown_2.7      pkgconfig_2.0.3   htmltools_0.5.1.1
[25] fastmap_1.1.0      rvg_0.2.5         htmlwidgets_1.5.3 rlang_0.4.10
[29] rstudioapi_0.13    shiny_1.6.0        generics_0.1.0    gamlss.data_5.1-4
[33] jsonlite_1.7.2     gtools_3.8.2       zip_2.1.1         magrittr_2.0.1
[37] Matrix_1.3-2       Rcpp_1.0.6         munsell_0.5.0     gdtools_0.2.3
[41] lifecycle_1.0.0    stringi_1.5.3      yaml_2.2.1        MASS_7.3-53.1
[45] gamlss.dist_5.1-7  grid_4.0.4         parallel_4.0.4   promises_1.2.0.1
[49] crayon_1.4.1       lattice_0.20-41    splines_4.0.4     hms_1.0.0
[53] pillar_1.4.7       uuid_0.1-4         glue_1.4.2        evaluate_0.14
[57] data.table_1.13.6  vctrs_0.3.6        httpuv_1.5.5      gtable_0.3.0
[61] purrr_0.3.4        assertthat_0.2.1   cachem_1.0.4      CDM_7.5-15
[65] xfun_0.21          mime_0.10          xtable_1.8-4      later_1.1.0.1
[69] survival_3.2-7     viridisLite_0.3.0  tibble_3.0.6      memoise_2.0.0
[73] ellipsis_0.3.1
```

Data availability

UNDERLYING DATA

The raw data needed to replicate these analyses are not public, so we cannot share it with this publication. However, the reader can apply for access to the data through the study contact. The table given below contains the contact information for each cohort included in this publication.

A subset of studies made their study data publicly available under a CC BY 4.0 license (https://creativecommons.org/licenses/by/4.0/)[1]. Authorship remains with the study coordinator, but users are free to redistribute, alter and combine the data, on the condition of giving appropriate credit with any redistributions of the material. The URL of the public data is https://d-score.org/childdevdata/.

Name in publication	Reference	Contact
GCDG-NLD-SMOCC	Herngreen *et al.*, 1992	Paul Verkerk (paul.verkerk@tno.nl)
TOGO	Van Buuren & Eekhout, 2021	Cécile Schat-Savy (cschatsavy@kinderhulp-togo.nl)
POPS	Verloove - Vanhorick *et al.*, 1986	Sylvia van de Pal (sylvia.vanderpal@tno.nl)

Note

1 Zenodo: D-score/childdevdata: childdevdata 1.0.1, http://doi.org/10.5281/zenodo.4685979 (van Buuren, 2021)

References

Andrich D: A Rating Formulation for Ordered Response Categories. *Psychometrika*. 1978; 43(4): 561–573. 10.1007/BF02293814

Baarda DB: *UKKI: Utrechtse Korte Kleuter Intelligentietest: Handleiding*. Lisse: Swets en Zeitlinger, 1978. Reference Source

Baird G, Simonoff E, Pickles A, *et al.*: Prevalence of Disorders of the Autism Spectrum in a Population Cohort of Children in South Thames: The Special Needs and Autism Project (SNAP).*Lancet*. 2006; 368(9531): 210–215. 1684449010.1016/S0140-6736(06)69041-7

Bellman M, Byrne O, Sege R: Developmental Assessment of Children. *BMJ*. 2013; 346 (e8687): e8687. 10.1136/bmj.e8687

Berk LE: *Child Development. 9th Ed.* Boston, MA: Pearson. 2011.

Berkson J: Application of the Logistic Function to Bio-Assay. *J Am Stat Assoc*. 1944; 39 (227): 357–365. 10.1080/01621459.1944.10500699

Black MM, Walker SP, Fernald LCH, *et al.*: Early Childhood Development Coming of Age: Science Through the Life Course. *Lancet*. 2017; 389(10064): 77–90. 2771761410.1016/S0140-6736(16)31389-75884058

Bock RD, Mislevy RJ: Adaptive EAP Estimation of Ability in a Microcomputer Environment. *Appl Psychol Meas*. 1982; 6(4): 431–444. 10.1177/014662168200600405

Boggs D, Milner KM, Chandna J, *et al.*: Rating Early Child Development Outcome Measurement Tools for Routine Health Programme Use. *Arch Dis Child*. 2019; 104(Suppl 1): S22–33. 3088596310.1136/archdischild-2018-3154316557219

Britto PR, Lye SJ, Proulx K, *et al.*: Nurturing Care: Promoting Early Childhood Development. *Lancet*. 2017; 389(10064): 91–102. 2771761510.1016/S0140-6736 (16)31390-3

Cameron N, Bogin B: *Human Growth and Development*. London: Academic Press, 2012. Reference Source

Caspi A, Hariri AR, Holmes A, *et al.*: Genetic Sensitivity to the Environment: The Case of the Serotonin Transporter Gene and Its Implications for Studying Complex Diseases and Traits. *Am J Psychiatry*. 2010; 167(5): 509–527. 2023132310.1176/appi.ajp.2010.091014522943341

Cole TJ: Fitting Smoothed Centile Curves to Reference Data (with Discussion). *J R Stat Soc Ser A*. 1988; 151(3): 385–418. 10.2307/2982992

Cole TJ, Green PJ: Smoothing Reference Centile Curves: The LMS Method and Penalized Likelihood. *Stat Med*. 1992; 11(10): 1305–1319. 151899210.1002/sim.4780111005

Coombs CH: *A Theory of Data*. New York: Wiley, 1964. Reference Source

Ellingsen KM: Standardized Assessment of Cognitive Development: Instruments and Issues. In *Early Childhood Assessment in School and Clinical Child Psychology*. edited by E. Garro, Springer, 2016; 25–49. 10.1007/978-1-4939-6349-2_2

Embretsen SE, Reise SP: *Item Response Theory for Psychologists*. Mahwah, NJ: Lawrence Erlbaum, 2000. Reference Source

Engelhard G: *Invariant Measurement*. New York: Routledge, 2013. Reference Source

Engle PL, Fernald LCH, Alderman H, *et al.*: Strategies for Reducing Inequalities and Improving Developmental Outcomes for Young Children in Low-Income and Middle-Income Countries. *Lancet.* 2011; 378(9799): 1339–1353. 2194437810.1016/S0140-6736(11)60889-1

Erikson EH: *Childhood and Society. 2d Ed., Rev. And Enl.* New York, NJ: Norton, 1963. Reference Source

Fernald LCH, Prado E, Kariger P, *et al.*: A Toolkit for Measuring Early Childhood Development in Low and Middle-Income Countries. 2017. Reference Source

Frankenburg WK, Dodds J, Archer P, *et al.*: The Denver II: A Major Revision and Restandardization of the Denver Developmental Screening Test. *Pediatrics.* 1992; 89(1): 91–97. 1370185

Gesell A: *Infant and Child in the Culture of Today.* Los Angeles, CA: Read Book Ltd, 1943. Reference Source

Grantham-McGregor SM, Fernald LCH, Kagawa RMC, *et al.*: Effects of Integrated Child Development and Nutrition Interventions on Child Development and Nutritional Status. *Ann N Y Acad Sci.* 2014; 1308(1): 11–32. 2467316610.1111/nyas.12284

Guttman L: The Basis for Scalogram Snalysis. In *Measurement and Prediction.* edited by S. A.StoufferL.GuttmanE. A.SuchmanP. F.LazarsfeldS. A.Star, and J. A. Clausen, Princeton, NJ: Princeton University Press, 1950; IV: 60–90.

Hafkamp-de Groen E, Dusseldorp E, Boere-Boonekamp MM, *et al.*: Relatie Tussen Het van Wiechenonderzoek (d-Score) Op 2 Jaar En Het Intelligentieniveau Op 5 Jaar. [relation Between the Dutch Development Instrument at the Age of 2 Years and Intelligence at the Age of 5 Years].*Tijdschrift Voor Jeugdgezondheidszorg.* 2009; 41(1): 10–13. Reference Source

Hattie J: Methodology Review: Assessing Unidimensionality of Tests and Itenls. *Appl Psychol Meas.* 1985; 9(2): 139–164. 10.1177/014662168500900204

Herngreen WP, Reerink JD, van Noord-Zaadstra BM, *et al.*: The SMOCC-study: Design of a representative cohort of live-born infants in the Netherlands. *Eur J Public Health.* 1992; 2(2): 117–122. 10.1093/eurpub/2.2.117

Herngreen WP, van Buuren S, van Wieringen JC, *et al.*: Growth in Length and Weight from Birth to 2 Years of a Representative Sample of Netherlands Children (born in 1988-89) Related to SocioEconomic Status and Other Background Characteristics. *Ann Hum Biol.* 1994; 21(5): 449–463. 798599410.1080/03014469400003472

Holland PW, Wainer H: *Differential Item Functioning.* Hillsdale, NJ: Lawrence Erlbaum Associates, 1983.

Horridge KA: Assessment and Investigation of the Child with Disordered Development. *Arch Dis Child Educ Pract Ed.* 2011; 96(1): 9–20. 2092662410.1136/adc.2009.182436

Jacobusse G, van Buuren S: Computerized Adaptive Testing for Measuring Development of Young Children. *Stat Med.* 2007; 26(13): 2629–2638. 1713364910.1002/sim.2753

Jacobusse G, van Buuren S, Verkerk PH: An Interval Scale for Development of Children Aged 0-2 Years. *Stat Med.* 2006; 25(13): 2272–2283. 1614399510.1002/sim.2351

Johnson SB, Riley AW, Granger DA, *et al.*: The Science of Early Life Toxic Stress for Pediatric Practice and Advocacy. *Pediatrics.* 2013; 131(2): 319–327. 2333922410.1542/peds.2012-04694074672

Kohlberg L: *The Psychology of Moral Development: The Nature and Validity of Moral Stages.* San Francisco: Harper & Row, 1984; 2. Reference Source

Kolb B, Harker A, Gibb R: Principles of Plasticity in the Developing Brain. *Dev Med Child Neurol.* 2017; 59(12): 1218–1223. 2890155010.1111/dmcn.13546

Liebert RM, Poulos RW, Strauss GD: *Developmental Psychology.* Englewood Cliffs, NJ: Prentice-Hall, Inc.1974. Reference Source

Linacre JM: Rasch Model Estimation: Further Topics. *J Appl Meas.* 2004; 5(1): 95–110. 14757994

Miller AC, Murray MB, Thomson DR, et al.: How Consistent Are Associations Between Stunting and Child Development? Evidence from a Meta-Analysis of Associations Between Stunting and Multidimensional Child Development in Fifteen Low- and Middle-Income Countries. *Public Health Nutr.* 2016; 19(8): 1339–1347. 2635542610.1017/S136898001500227X

Mokken RJ: *A Theory and Procedure of Scale Analysis: With Applications in Political Research.* Berlin: Walter de Gruyter, 1971. 10.1515/9783110813203

Molenaar IW: Nonparametric Models for Polytomous Responses. In *Handbook of Modern Item Response Theory.* Springer, 1997; 369–380. 10.1007/978-1-4757-2691-6_21

Perkins JM, Kim R, Krishna A, et al.: Understanding the Association Between Stunting and Child Development in Low- and Middle-Income Countries: Next Steps for Research and Intervention. *Soc Sci Med.* 2017; 193: 101–109. 2902855710.1016/j.socscimed.2017.09.039

Piaget J, Inhelder B: *The Psychology of the Child.* New York, NJ: Basic Books, 1969. Reference Source

Rasch G: *Probabilistic Models for Some Intelligence and Attainment Tests.* Copenhagen: Danish Institute for Educational Research. 1960. Reference Source

Rasch G: On Specific Objectivity: An Attempt at Formalizing the Request for Generality and Validity of Scientific Statements. *The Danish Yearbook of Philosophy.* 1977; 14: 58–93. Reference Source

Robitzsch A: Sirt: Supplementary Item Response Theory Models. 2016. Reference Source

Rutter M: Genes and Behavior: Nature-Nurture Interplay Explained. Hogrefe Publishing, 2007.

Salkind NJ: Child Development. Macmillan Library Reference, 2002. Reference Source

Santrock JW: *Child Development: An Introduction. 13th Ed.* New York, NJ: McGraw-Hill Higher Education, 2011. Reference Source

Shirley MM: *The First Two Years: A Study of Twenty-Five Babies. Vol. I: Postural and Locomotor Development.* Minneapolis: University of Minnesota Press, 1931. Reference Source

Shirley MM: *The First Two Years: A Study of Twenty-Five Babies. Vol. II: Intellectual Development.* Minneapolis: University of Minnesota Press, 1933.

Shonkhoff JP, Levitt P, Fox NA, et al.: From Best Practices to Breakthrough Impacts: A Science-Based Approach to Building a More Promising Future for Young Children and Families. Harvard University, Center on the Developing Child Cambridge, MA. 2016. Reference Source

Stasinopoulos DM, Rigby RA: Generalized Additive Models for Location Scale and Shape (GAMLSS) in r. *J Stat Softw.* 2008; 23(7): 1–46. 10.18637/jss.v023.i07

Stott LH: *Child Development: An Individual Longitudinal Approach.* New York, NJ: Holt, Rinehart; Winston, Inc. 1967. 10.1002/1520-6807(196801)5:1<92::AID-PITS2310050120>3.0.CO;2-D

Sudfeld CR, McCoy DC, Danaei G, *et al.*: Linear Growth and Child Development in Low- and Middle-Income Countries: A Meta-Analysis. *Pediatrics.* 2015; 135(5): e1266–75. 2584780610.1542/peds.2014-3111

van Buuren S: Growth Charts of Human Development. *Stat Methods Med Res.* 2014; 23 (4): 346–368. 2348701910.1177/0962280212473300

van Buuren S: D-score/childdevdata: childdevdata 1.0.1. (Version v1.0.1).*Zenodo.* 2021. http://www.doi.org/10.5281/zenodo.4685979

van Buuren S, Eekhout I: Child development with the D-score: tuning instruments to unity. *F1000Res.* (in press). 2021. Reference Source

Verloove-Vanhorick SP, Verwey RA, Brand R, *et al.*: Neonatal Mortality Risk in Relation to Gestational Age and Birthweight. Results of a National Survey of Preterm and Very-Low-Birthweight Infants in the Netherlands. *Lancet.* 1986; 1 (8472): 55–57. 286731210.1016/s0140-6736(86)90713-0

Vlasblom E, Boere-Boonekamp MM, Hafkamp-de Groen E, *et al.*: Predictive Validity of Developmental Milestones for Detecting Limited Intellectual Functioning. *PLoS One.* 2019; 14(3): e0214475. 3092142410.1371/journal.pone.02144756438572

Wainer H, Dorans NJ, Flaugher R, *et al.*: Computerized Adaptive Testing: A Primer. Routledge, 2000. Reference Source

Wit JM, Himes JH, van Buuren S, *et al.*: Practical Application of Linear Growth Measurements in Clinical Research in Low- and Middle-Income Countries. *Horm Res Paediatr.* 2017; 88(1): 79–90. 2819636210.1159/0004560075804842

Wright BD, Masters GN: *Rating Scale Analysis: Rasch Measurement.* Chicago: MESA Press, 1982. Reference Source

Zumbo BD: A Handbook on the Theory and Methods of Differential Item Functioning (DIF).*Ottawa: National Defense Headquarters.* 1999. Reference Source

Zwinderman AH: Pairwise Parameter Estimation in Rasch Models. *Appl Psychol Meas.* 1995; 19(4): 369–375. 10.1177/014662169501900406

2

Child development with the D-score: tuning instruments to unity

Edited by
Iris Eekhout[1] and Stef van Buuren[1,2]
[1]Netherlands Organisation for Applied Scientific Research TNO, Leiden, 2316 ZL, The Netherlands
[2]University of Utrecht, Utrecht, 3584 CH, The Netherlands

2.1 Introduction

Iris Eekhout[1]
Stef van Buuren[1,2]
[1]Netherlands Organisation for Applied Scientific Research TNO, Leiden, 2316 ZL, The Netherlands
[2]University of Utrecht, Utrecht, 3584 CH, The Netherlands

This introductory section

- briefly summarizes our previous work on the D-score (2.1.1)
- introduces the main topic of the chapter (2.1.2)
- highlights the relevance of work (2.1.3)
- explains why we have written this chapter (2.1.4)
- delineates the intended audience (2.1.5)

2.1.1 PREVIOUS WORK ON THE D-SCORE

Chapter 1 highlighted the concepts and tools needed to obtain a quantitative score from a set of developmental milestones.

In practice, we typically want to make the following types of comparisons:

- Compare development within the same child over time;
- Compare the development of two children of the same age;
- Compare the development of two children of different ages;
- Compare the development of groups of children of different ages.

To do this well, we need an *interval scale with a fixed unit of development*. We argued that the simple Rasch model is a very suitable candidate to provide us with such a unit. The Rasch model is simple, fast, and we found that it fits child developmental data very well (Jacobusse *et al.*, 2006; van Buuren, 2014). The Rasch model has a long history, but (unfortunately) it is almost unknown outside the field of psychometrics. We highlighted the concepts of the model that are of direct relevance to child development. Using data collected by the Dutch Development Instrument, we demonstrated that the model and its estimates behave as intended for children in the open population, for prematurely born-children, and children living in a low- and middle-income country.

As our approach breaks with the traditional paradigm that emphasizes different domains of child development, we expected a slow uphill battle for acceptance. We have now gained the interest from various prominent authors in

DOI: 10.1201/9781003216315-12

the field, and from organizations who recognize the value of a one-number-summary for child development. In analogy to traditional growth charts, it is entirely possible to track children, or groups of children, on a developmental chart over time. Those and other applications of the technology may eventually win over some more souls.

2.1.2 WHAT THIS VOLUME IS ABOUT

It is straightforward to apply the D-score methodology, as explained in Chapter 1: Turning milestones into measurement (van Buuren & Eekhout, 2021), for measurements observed by one instrument. In practice, however, there is a complication. We often need to deal with multiple, partially overlapping tools. For example, our data may contain

- different versions of the same instrument (e.g., Bayley I, II and III);
- different language versions of the same tool;
- different tools administered to the same sample;
- different tools administered to different samples;
- and so on.

Since there are over 150 different instruments to measure child development (Fernald *et al.*, 2017), the chances are high that our data also hold data observed by multiple tools.

It is not apparent how to obtain comparable scores from different instruments. Tools may have idiosyncratic instructions to calculate total scores, distinctive domain definitions, unique compositions of norm groups, different floors and ceilings, or combinations of these.

This chapter addresses the problem *how to define and calculate the D-score based on data coming from multiple sources, using various instruments administered at varying ages.* We explain techniques that systematically exploit the overlap between tools to create comparable scores. For example, many instruments have variations on milestones like *Can stack two blocks, Can stand* or *Says baba.* By carefully mapping out the similarities between instruments, we can construct a constrained measurement model informed by subject matter knowledge. As a result, we can map different instruments onto the same scale.

Many of the techniques are well known within psychometrics and educational research. This chapter translates the concepts to the field of child development.

2.1.3 RELEVANCE OF THE WORK

We all like our children to grow and prosper. The *first 1000 days* refers to the time needed for a child to grow from conception to its second birthday. During this period, the architecture of the developing brain is very open to the influence of relationships and experiences. It is a time of rapid change that lays the groundwork for later health and happiness.

Professionals and parents consider it necessary to monitor children's development. While we can track the child's physical growth by growth charts to identify children with signs of potential delay, there are no charts for monitoring child development. To create such charts, we need to have a unit of development, similar to units like centimetres or kilograms.

The D-score is a way to define a unit of child development. With the D-score, we see that progress is much faster during infancy, and that different children develop at different rates. The D-score also allows us to define a "normal" range that we can use to filter out those who are following a more pathological course. There is good evidence that early identification and early intervention improve the outcomes of children (Britto *et al.*, 2017). Early intervention is crucial for children with developmental disabilities because barriers to healthy development early in life impede progress at each subsequent stage.

Monitoring child development provides caregivers and parents with reliable information about the child and an opportunity to intervene at an early age. Understanding the developmental health of populations of children allows organizations and policymakers to make informed decisions about programmes that support children's greatest needs (Bellman *et al.*, 2013).

2.1.4   WHY THIS CHAPTER?

We believe that *there can be one scale* for measuring child development and that this scale is useful for many applications. We also believe that *there cannot be one instrument* for measuring child development that is suitable for all situations. In general, the tool needs tailoring to the setting.

We see that practitioners often view instruments and scales as exchangeable. In daily practice, the practitioner would pick a particular tool to measure a specific faculty, which then effectively produces a "scale score." Each tool produces its own score, which then feeds into the diagnostic and monitoring process.

We have always found it difficult to explain that scales and instruments are different things. For us, a scale is a continuous concept, like "distance," "temperature" or "child development," and the instrument is the way to assign values to the particular object being measured. For measuring distance, we use devices like rods, tapes, sonar, radar, geo-location, or red-shift detection, and we can express the results as the location under the underlying scale (e.g., number of meters). It would undoubtedly be an advance if we could establish a *unit of child development*, and express the measurement as the number of units. If we succeed, we can compare child development scores, that are measured through different devices. This chapter explores the theory and practice for making that happen.

2.1.5   INTENDED AUDIENCE

We aim for three broad audiences:

- Professionals in the field of child growth and development;
- Policymakers in international settings;
- Statisticians, methodologists, and data scientists.

Professionals in child development are constantly faced with the problem that different instruments for measuring child development yield incomparable scores. This chapter introduces and illustrates sound psychometric techniques *for extracting comparable scores from existing instruments*. We hope that our approach will ease communication between professionals.

Policymakers in international settings are looking for simple, versatile, and cheap instruments to gain insight into the effectiveness of interventions. The ability to measure child development by a single number *enhances priority setting and leads to a more accurate understanding of policy effects*.

The text may appeal to statisticians and data scientists for *the simplicity of the concepts, for the (somewhat unusual) application of statistical models to discard data, for the ease of interpretation of the result, and for the availability of software*.

2.2 Data

Iris Eekhout[1]
Stef van Buuren[1,2]
[1]Netherlands Organisation for Applied Scientific
Research TNO, Leiden, 2316 ZL, The Netherlands
[2]University of Utrecht, Utrecht, 3584 CH, The
Netherlands

This chapter explains the methodology for obtaining a comparable developmental score (D-score) from different instruments. This section introduces the data that will illustrate our approach. The data originates from a study by the Global Child Development Group (GCDG), that brought together longitudinal measurement on child development data from 16 cohorts worldwide.

- Overview of cohorts and instrument (2.2.1)
- Cohort descriptions (2.2.2)
- Instruments (2.2.3)

2.2.1 OVERVIEW OF COHORTS AND INSTRUMENTS

The Global Child Development Group (GCDG) collected longitudinal data from 16 cohorts. The objective of the study was to develop a population-based measure to monitor early child development across ages and countries. The requirements for inclusion were

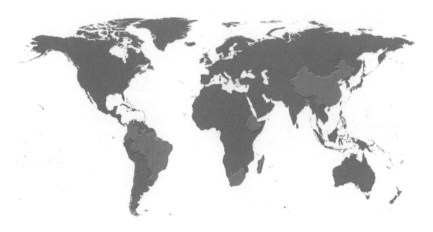

FIGURE 2.2.1 Coverage of countries included in the study.

DOI: 10.1201/9781003216315-13

1. direct assessment of child development;
2. availability of individual milestone scores;
3. spanning ages between 0–5 years;
4. availability of follow-up measures, at ages 5–10 years.

The effort resulted in a database containing individual data from over 16,000 children from 11 countries. The world map shown in Figure 2.2.1 colors the countries included in the study. Section 2.2.2 briefly describes each cohort. Section 2.2.3 reviews the measurement instruments.

The GCDG data consists of birth cohorts, impact evaluation studies and instrument evaluation studies.

2.2.2   COHORT DESCRIPTIONS

The cohorts have different designs, age ranges and assessment instruments. Figure 2.2.2 displays the age range of developmental assessments per cohort, coloured according to the instruments.

A brief description of each cohort follows:

The **Bangladesh** study (GCDG-BGD-7MO) was an impact evaluation study including 1862 children around the age of 18 months. The Bayley Scale for Infant and Toddler Development-II (by2) was administered and long-term follow-up data were available for the Wechsler Preschool and Primary Scale of Intelligence (WPPSI) at 5 years (Tofail *et al.*, 2008).

The **Brazil 1** study (GCDG-BRA-1) was a birth-cohort with 3 measurement moments: 644 children at 3 months, 1412 children at 6 months and 1362 children at 12 months. The investigators administered the Denver Developmental Screening Test-II (den) in each round. Long-term follow-up data were

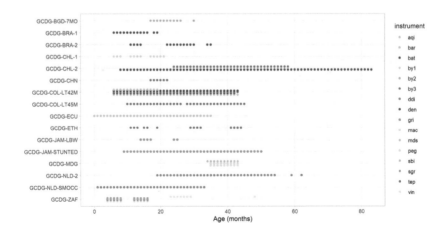

FIGURE 2.2.2   Age range and assessment instrument of included data for each GCDG cohort.

available for the Wechsler Adult Intelligence Scale (WAIS) at 18 years (Victora *et al.*, 2006).

The **Brazil 2** study (GCDG-BRA-2) was a birth-cohort with measurements of 3907 children at 12 months and 3869 children at 24 months. Both occasions collected data on the Battelle Development Inventory (bat) (Moura *et al.*, 2010).

The **Chile 1** study (GCDG-CHL-1) was an impact evaluation study of 128 children assessed at 6 months, 1732 children at 12 months and 279 at 18 months. The by1 was administered at each of the three waves. Long-term follow-up data were available for the WPPSI at 5–6 years (Lozoff *et al.*, 2003).

The **Chile 2** study (GCDG-CHL-2) consists of a birth-cohort of 4869 children. The investigators measured child development by the Battelle Developmental Inventory (bat) at 7–23 months. A total of 9201 children aged 24–58 responded to the Test de Desarrollo Psicomotor (tep) at 24–58 months. For the latter group, follow-up data were available for the Peabody Picture Vocabulary Test (PPVT) at 5–6 years (Conteras & González, 2015).

The **China** study (GCDG-CHN) was an impact evaluation study that contained 990 children assessed with the by3 at 18 months (Lozoff *et al.*, 2016).

The **Colombia 1** study (GCDG-COL-LT45M) was an impact evaluation study that comprised two waves. Wave 1 contained 704 children at 12–24 months and wave 2 631 children at 24–41 months. The by3 was administered at each wave. Long-term follow-up data were available for PPVT at 4–6 years (Attanasio *et al.*, 2014).

The **Colombia 2** study (GCDG-COL-LT42M) was an instrument validation study where all 1311 children aged 6–42 months were measured the by3. Also, there are data for a subgroup of 658 children on den, the Ages and Stages Questionnaire (aqi), and the bat screener. Long-term follow-up data were available for the Fifth Wechsler Intelligence Scale for Children (WISC-V) and the PPVT (Rubio-Codina *et al.*, 2016).

An impact evaluation study in **Ecuador** (GCDG-ECU) yielded data from 667 children between 0–35 months on the Barrera Moncada (bar). Long-term follow-up data were available for the PPVT at 5–8 and 9–12 years [Paxson & Schady, 2010].

The **Ethiopia** study (GCDG-ETH) was a birth-cohort with 193 children of 12 months in the first wave, 440 children of 30 months at the second wave, and 456 children of 42 months at the third wave. The investigators used the same instrument (by3) for all waves. Long-term follow-up data were available for the PPVT at 10–11 years [Hanlon *et al.*, 2009].

The **Jamaica 1** study (GCDG-JAM-LBW) was an impact evaluation study that collected data on the Griffiths Mental Development Scales (gri) for 225 children aged 15 months (first wave), and 218 children of aged 24 months (second wave). Long-term follow-up data were available for WPPSI and PPVT at 6 years (Walker *et al.*, 2004).

The **Jamaica 2** study (GCDG-JAM-STUNTED) was an impact evaluation study with data on the gri for 159 children at 9–24 months, 21–36 months, and at 33–48 months. Long-term follow-up data were available for sbi, Raven's Coloured Progressive Matrices (Ravens), and PPVT at 7–8 years and the WAIS at 17–18 years (Grantham-McGregor *et al.*, 1991).

The **Madagascar** study (GCDG-MDG) was an impact evaluation study that used the sbi for 205 children aged 34–42 months. Long-term follow-up data were available for sbi and PPVT at 7–11 years (Fernald *et al.*, 2011).

The **Netherlands 1** study (GCDG-NLD-SMOCC) was an instrument validation study with a total of 9 waves. At each wave the Dutch Developmental instrument (ddi) (In the Netherlands known as Van Wiechenschema) was administered. The first wave included 1985 children at 1 month, wave 2 1807 children at 2 months, wave 3 1963 children at 3 months, wave 4 1919 children at 6 months, wave 5 1881 children at 9 months, wave 6 1802 children at 12 months, wave 7 1776 children at 15 months, wave 8 1787 children at 18 months, and wave 9 1815 children at 24 months (Herngreen *et al.*, 1992).

The **Netherlands 2** study (GCDG-NLD-2) was an instrument validation study with a total of five waves. This study resembles GCDG-NLD-SMOCC but for older children. Wave 1 included 1016 children at 24 months, wave 2 995 children at 30 months, wave 3 1592 children at 36 months, wave 4 1592 children at 42 months, and wave 5 1024 children at 48 months (Doove, 2010).

The **South Africa** study (GCDG-ZAF) was a birth cohort with four waves. The first wave included 485 children and second wave 275 children, who were assessed at 6 and 12 months, respectively, with the by1 and the gri. The third wave included 1802 children and the fourth wave 1614 children, assessed at 24 and 48 months, respectively, with the Vineland Social Maturity Scale (vin) (Richter *et al.*, 2007).

2.2.3 INSTRUMENTS

The **Bayley Scales for Infant and Toddler Development** (by1, by2, by3) aim to assess infants and toddlers, aged 1–42 months. The current version is the by3, but some GCDG cohorts used earlier versions (i.e. by1 and by2) (Bayley, 1969; Bayley, 1993; Bayley, 2006). The 326 items of the by3 measure three domains: Cognitive items, Motor items (with fine and gross motor items), and Language items (with expressive and receptive items). The by2 contains 277 items and has two additional subscales: Social-Emotional and Adaptive Behavior. by1 contains 229 items.

The **Denver Developmental Screening Test** (den) is aimed to identify developmental problems in children up to age six. The 125 dichotomous test items are distributed over the age range from birth to six years. The Denver covers four domains: personal-social, fine motor and adaptive, language, and gross motor. The test items are all directly observed by an examiner and are not dependent on parent report (Frankenburg *et al.*, 1992) (Frankenburg *et al.*, 1990).

The **Griffiths Mental Development Scales** (gri) measure the rate of development in infants and young children in six developmental areas:

locomotor, personal-social, hearing and language, eye and hand coordination, performance and practical reasoning (Griffiths, 1967).

The **Battelle Developmental Inventory** (bat) measures key developmental skills in children from birth to 7 years, 11 months. The instrument contains 450 items distributed over five domains: adaptive, personal-social, communication, motor, and cognitive (Newborg, 2005).

The **Vineland Social Maturity Scale** (vin) is a test to assess social competence. The instrument contains eight subscales that measure communication skills, general self-help ability, locomotion skills, occupation skills, self-direction, self-help eating, self-help dressing and socialization skills (Doll, 1953).

The **Dutch Developmental Instrument** (ddi) measures early child development during the ages 0–4 years. The instrument consists of 75 milestones spread over three domains: fine motor, adaptive, personal and social behaviour; communication; and gross motor (Schlesinger-Was, 1981).

The **Barrera Moncada** (bar) is a Spanish instrument that measures the growth and psychological development of children (Moncada, 1981).

The **Test de Desarrollo Psicomotor** (tep) is an instrument to evaluate toddlers aged 2 to 5 years on their development. The items come from three sub-tests: 16 items assess coordination; 24 items measure language skills and 12 items tap into motor skills (Haeussler & Marchant, 1999).

The **Ages and Stages Questionnaire** (aqi) measures developmental progress in children aged 2 mo – 5.5 yrs. The instrument distinguishes development in five areas: personal-social, gross motor, fine motor, problem solving, and communication. The caregiver completes 30 items per age intervals and (Squires & Bricker, 2009).

The **Stanford Binet Intelligence Scales** (sbi) is a cognitive ability and intelligence test to diagnose developmental deficiencies in young children. The items divide into five subtests: fluid reasoning, knowledge, quantitative reasoning, visual-spatial processing, and working memory (Roid, 2003) (Hagen & Stattler, 1986).

2.3 Comparability

Iris Eekhout[1]
Stef van Buuren[1,2]
[1]Netherlands Organisation for Applied Scientific Research TNO, Leiden, 2316 ZL, The Netherlands
[2]University of Utrecht, Utrecht, 3584 CH, The Netherlands

This section describes challenges and methodologies to harmonize child development measurements obtained by different instruments:

- Are instruments connected? (2.3.1)
- Bridging instruments by mapping items (2.3.2)
- Overview of promising item mappings (2.3.3)

2.3.1 ARE INSTRUMENTS CONNECTED?

The ultimate goal is to compare child development across populations and cultures. A complication is that measurements are made by different instruments. To do deal with this issue, we harmonize the data included in the GCDG cohorts. In particular, we process the milestone responses such that the following requirements hold:

- Every milestone in an instrument has a unique name and a descriptive label;
- Every milestone occupies one column in the dataset;
- Item scores are (re)coded as: 1 = PASS; 0 = FAIL;
- Items not administered or not answered are a missing value;
- Every row in the dataset corresponds to a unique cohort-child-age combination.
- Two cohorts are indirectly connected if both connect to a third cohort that connects them.
- Two instruments are indirectly connected if both connect to a third instrument that connects them.
- Any differences between studies can be attributed to the difficulties of the instruments.

Cohorts and milestones need to be *connected*. There are several ways to connect cohorts:

- Two cohorts are directly connected if they use the same instrument;

DOI: 10.1201/9781003216315-14

- Two cohorts are indirectly connected if both connect to a third cohort that connects them.
- Two instruments are indirectly connected if both connect to a third instrument that connects them.
- Any differences between studies can be attributed to the difficulties of the instruments.

Likewise, instruments can be connected:

- Two instruments are directly connected if the same cohort measures both;
- Two instruments are indirectly connected if both connect to a third instrument that connects them.
- Any differences between studies can be attributed to the difficulties of the instruments.

An X in Table 2.3.1 identifies which cohorts use which instruments. The linkage table shows that studies from China, Colombia, and Ethiopia are directly connected (by by3). Brazil 1 indirectly connects to these studies through den. Some cohorts (e.g., Chile 1 and Ecuador) do not link to any other study. Likewise, we might say that aqi, bat, by3, and den are directly connected. Note that no indirect connections exist to this instrument group.

Table 2.3.1 is a somewhat simplified version of the linkage pattern. As we saw in section 2.2.2, there are substantial age differences between the cohorts. The linked instrument linkage table shows the counts of the number of registered scores per age group. What appears in Table 2.3.1 as one test may consist of two disjoint subsets, and hence some cohorts may not be connected after all.

Connectedness is a necessary - though not sufficient - requirement for parameter identification. If two cohorts are not connected, we cannot distinguish between the following two alternative explanations:

- Any differences between studies can be attributed to the ability of the children;
- Any differences between studies can be attributed to the difficulties of the instruments.

The data do not contain the necessary information to discriminate between these two explanations. Since many cohorts in Table 2.3.1 are unconnected, it seems that we are stuck.

The next section suggests a way out of the dilemma.

2.3.2   BRIDGING INSTRUMENTS BY MAPPING ITEMS

Many instruments for measuring child development have appeared since the works of Shirley (1933) and Gesell (1943). It is no surprise that their contents

TABLE 2.3.1

Linkage pattern indicating combinations of cohorts and instruments.

	aqi	bar	bat	by1	by2	by3	ddi	den	gri	mac	peg	sbi	sgr	tep	vin
Bangladesh					x										
Brazil 1								x							
Brazil 2			x												
Chile 1				x											
Chile 2			x											x	
China						x									
Colombia 1						x									
Colombia 2	x		x			x		x							
Ecuador		x													
Ethiopia						x									
Jamaica 1									x						
Jamaica 2									x						
Madagascar										x	x	x			
Netherlands1							x								
Netherlands2							x		x						
South Africa					x				x				x		x

show substantial overlap. All tools assess events like starting to see, hear, smile, fetch, crawl, walk, speak, and think. We will exploit this overlap to bridge different instruments. For example, Table 2.3.2 displays the labels of milestones from six instruments. All items probe the ability of the child to formulate "sentences" of two words.

The idea is to check whether these milestones measure development in the same way. If this is found to be true, then we may formally restrict the

---

TABLE 2.3.2

Example of similar items from different instruments.

Item	Label
by1mdd136	Sentence of 2 words
by2mdd114	Uses a two-word utterance
ddicmm041	Says sentences with 2 words
denlgd019	Combine Words
grihsd217	Uses word combinations
vinxxc016	Use a short sentence

 Fine Motor Domain

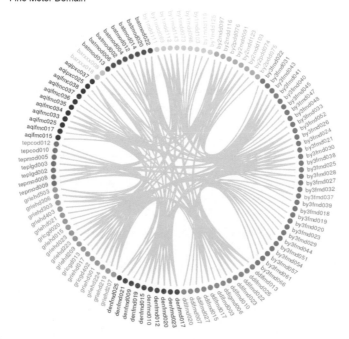

FIGURE 2.3.1 Connections between the instruments via mapped item groups for the fine motor domain (https://tnochildhealthstatistics.shinyapps.io/GCDG_mapping/).

difficulty levels of these milestones to be identical. This restriction provides a formal bridge between the instruments. We repeat the process for all groups of similar-looking items.

A first step in the bridging process is to group items from different instruments by similarity. As the by3 is relatively long and is the most often used instrument, it provides a convenient starting point. Subject matter experts experienced in child development mapped items from other tools to by3 items. These experts evaluated the similarity of wordings and descriptions in reference manuals. Also, they mapped same-skill items across other instruments into groups if these did not map onto by3 items.

Figure 2.3.1 connects similar items and hence visualizes connections between instruments for the fine motor domain. Items are displayed in the wheel, coloured by instrument. In the online application we organized item mappings into five domains: fine motor (FM), gross motor (GM), cognitive (COG), receptive (REC), and expressive (EXP). The Prev and Next buttons allow us to visit other domains.

2.3.3   AGE PROFILE OF ITEM MAPPINGS

Another way to explore the similarity of milestones from different instruments is to plot the probability of passing by age. Figure 2.3.2 shows two examples. The first graph presents the age curves of a group of four cognitive items for assessing the ability to put a cube or block in a cup or box. The milestones are administered in different studies and seem to work similarly. The second plot shows a similar graph for items that assess the ability to build a tower of six cubes or blocks. These milestones have similar age patterns as well.

Figure 2.3.3 presents two examples of weak item mappings. Notable timing differences exist for the "babbles" and "bangs" milestones, which suggests that we should not take these as bridges.

While these plots are suggestive, their interpretation is surprisingly complicated. We may find that age profiles of two milestones *A and B* administered in samples 1 and 2, respectively, *are identical* if

- A and B are equally difficult and samples 1 and 2 have the same maturation level;
- A is more difficult than B and sample 1 is more advanced than 2.

Similarly, we may find that the age profile for *A is earlier than B* if

- A is easier than B and if samples 1 and 2 have the same level of maturation;
- A and B are equally difficult and if sample 1 is more advanced than sample 2.

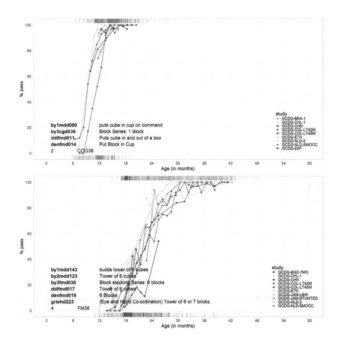

FIGURE 2.3.2 The probability of passing by age in potential bridging items.

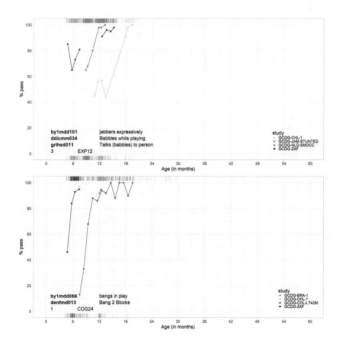

FIGURE 2.3.3 Probability to pass items for age in poor bridges.

Note that the age curves confound difficulty and ability, and hence cannot be used to evaluate the quality of the item map.

What we need to do is separate difficulty and ability. For this, we need a formal statistical model. The next section introduces the concepts required in such a model.

2.4 Equate groups

Iris Eekhout[1]
Stef van Buuren[1,2]
[1]Netherlands Organisation for Applied Scientific Research TNO, Leiden, 2316 ZL, The Netherlands
[2]University of Utrecht, Utrecht, 3584 CH, The Netherlands

This section introduces the concepts and tools needed to link assessments made by different instruments administered across multiple cohorts. Our methodology introduces the idea of an equate group. Systematic application of equate groups provides a robust yet flexible methodology to link different instruments. Once the links are in place, we may combine the data to enable meta-analyses and related methods.

- What is an equate group? (2.4.1)
- Concurrent calibration (2.4.2)
- Strategy to form and test equate groups (2.4.3)
- Statistical framework (2.4.4)
- Common latent scale (2.4.5)
- Quantifying equate fit (2.4.6)
- Differential item functioning (2.4.7)

2.4.1 WHAT IS AN EQUATE GROUP?

An *equate group* is a set of two or more milestones that measure the same thing in (perhaps slightly) different ways. Table 2.3.2 contains an example of an equate group, containing items that measure the ability to form two-word sentences. Also, Figure 2.3.2 and Figure 2.3.3 show examples of equate groups.

Equate groups vary in quality. We can use high-quality equate groups to link instruments by restricting the difficulty of all milestones in the equate group to be identical. Equate groups thus provide a method for bridging different tools.

Figure 2.4.1 displays items from three different instruments with overlapping sets of milestones. The shared items make up equate groups, as presented by the arrows between them. In the example, all three instruments share one milestone ("walk alone"). The "sitting" and "clap hand" items appear in two tools. So in total, there are three equate groups.

DOI: 10.1201/9781003216315-15

2.4.2 CONCURRENT CALIBRATION

Patterns as in Figure 2.4.1 occur if we have multiple forms of the same instrument. Although in theory, there might be sequence effects, the usual working assumption is that we may ignore them. Equate groups with truly shared items that work in the same way across samples are of high quality. We may collect the responses on identical items into the same column of the data matrix. As a consequence, usual estimation methods will automatically produce one difficulty estimate for that column (i.e. common item).

The procedure described above is known as *concurrent calibration*. See Kim & Cohen (1998) for more background. The method simultaneously estimates the item parameters for all instruments. Concurrent calibration is an attractive option for various reasons:

- It yields a common latent scale across all instruments;
- It is efficient because it calibrates all items in a single run;
- It produces more stable estimates for common items in small samples.

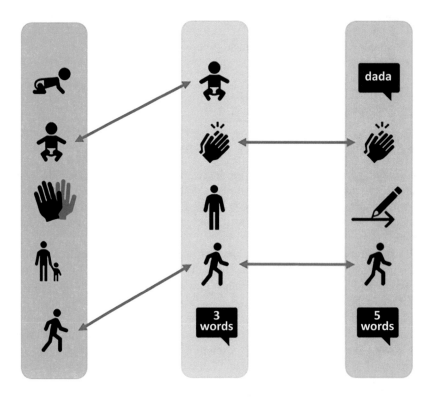

FIGURE 2.4.1   Example of three instruments that are bridged by common items in equate groups.

However, concurrent calibration depends on a strict distinction between items that are indeed the same across instruments and items that differ.

In practice, strict black-white distinctions may not be possible. Items that measure the same skill may have been adapted to suit the format of the instrument (e.g. number of response options, question formulation, and so on). Also, investigators may have altered the item to suit the local language and cultural context. Such changes may or may not affect the measurement properties. The challenge is to find out whether items measure the underlying construct in the same way.

In practice, we may need to perform concurrent calibration to multiple - perhaps slightly dissimilar - milestones. When confronted with similar - but not identical - items, our strategy is first to form provisional equate groups. We then explore, test and rearrange these equate groups, in the hope of finding enough high-quality equate groups that will bridge instruments.

2.4.3   STRATEGY TO FORM AND TEST EQUATE GROUPS

An equate group is a collection of items. Content matter experts may form equate groups by evaluating the contents of items and organizing them into groups with similar meaning. The modelling phase takes this set of equate groups (which may be hundreds) as input. Based on the analytic result, we may activate or modify equate groups. It is useful to distinguish between *active* and *passive* equate groups. What do we mean by these terms?

- *Active equate group*: The analysis treats all items within an active equate group as one super-item. The items obtain the same difficulty estimate and are assumed to yield equivalent measurements. As the items in an active equate group may originate from different instruments, such a group acts as a bridge between instruments.
- *Passive equate group*: Any non-active equate groups are called passive. The model does not restrict the difficulty estimates, i.e., the milestones within a passive equate group will have separate difficulty estimates.

Since active equate groups bridge different instruments, they have an essential role in the analysis. In general, we will set the status of an equate group to active *only* if we believe that the milestones in that group measure the underlying construct in the same way. Note that this does not necessarily imply that all items need to be identical. In Table 2.3.2, for example, small differences exist in item formulation. We may nevertheless believe that these are irrelevant and ignore these in practice. Reversely, there is no guarantee that the same milestone will measure child development in the same way in different samples. For example, a milestone like "climb stairs" (Figure 2.4.2) could be more difficult (and more dangerous) for children who have never seen a staircase.

The data analysis informs decisions to activate equate groups. The following steps implement our strategy for forming and enabling equate groups:

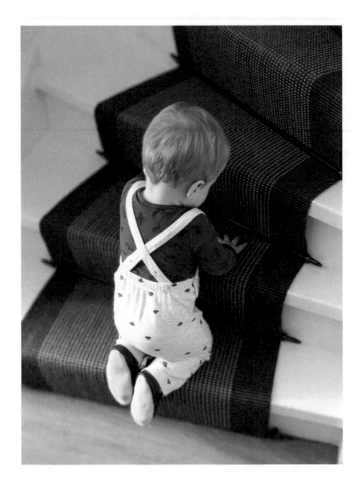

FIGURE 2.4.2   One year old child climbs stairs.

Photo by Iris Eekhout.

- Content matter experts compare milestones from different instruments and sort similar milestones into equate groups. It may be convenient to select one instrument as a starting point, and map items from others to that (see section 2.3.2);
- Visualize age profiles of mapped items (see section 2.3.3). Verify the plausibility of potential matches through similar age profiles. Break up mappings for which age profiles appear implausible. This step requires both statistical and subject matter expertise;
- Fit the model to the data using a subset of equate groups as active. Review the quality of the solution and optimize the quality of the links between tools by editing the equate group structure. The technical details

of this model are explained in section 2.4.4. Refit the model until (1) active equate groups link all cohorts and instruments, (2) active equate groups are distributed over the full-scale range (rather than being centred at one point);

- Assess the quality of equate groups by the infit and outfit (see section 2.4.6).
- Test performance of the equate groups across subgroups or cohorts by methods designed to detect differential item functioning (see section 2.4.7).

The application of equate groups is needed to connect different instruments to a universal scale. The technique is especially helpful in the situation where abilities differ across cohorts.

If the cohort abilities are relatively uniform (for example as a result of experimental design) and if the risk of misspecification of the equate groups is high, a good alternative is to rely on the equality of ability distribution. In our application, this was not an option due to the substantial age variation between cohorts.

2.4.4   PARAMETER ESTIMATION WITH EQUATE GROUPS

The Rasch model is the preferred measurement model for child development data. Section 1.4 provides an introduction of the Rasch model geared towards the D-score.

The Rasch model expresses the probability of passing an item as a logistic function of the difference between the person ability β_n and the item difficulty δ_i. The model (2.4.1) is defined as

$$\pi_{ni} = \frac{\exp (\beta_n - \delta_i)}{1 + \exp (\beta_n - \delta_i)}$$

Formula 2.4.1.

One way to interpret the formula is as follows. The logarithm of the odds that a person with ability β_n passes an item of difficulty δ_i is equal to the difference $\beta_i - \delta_i$ (Wright & Masters, 1982). See the logistic model in Section 1. 4.6.1 for more detail.

In model (2.4.1) every milestone i has one parameter δ_i. We extend the Rasch model by restricting the δ_i of all items within the same equate group to the same value. We thereby effectively say that these items are interchangeable measures of child development.

Estimation of the parameter for the equate group is straightforward. Wright & Masters (1982) present a simple method for aligning two test forms with common items. There are three steps:

- Estimate the separate δ_i's per item;
- Combine these estimates into δ_q by calculating their weighted average;
- Overwrite each δ_i by δ_q.

TABLE 2.4.1

Overview of the symbols used in equations (2.4.1) and (2.4.2).

Symbol	Term	Description
β_n	Ability	True (but unknown) developmental score of child n
δ_i	Difficulty	True (but unknown) difficulty of item i
δ_q	Difficulty	The combined difficulty of the items in equate group q
π_{ni}	Probability	Probability that child n passes item i
l		The number of items in the equate group
w_i		The number of respondents with an observed score on item i

Suppose that Q is the collection of items in equate group q, and that w_i is the number of respondents for item i. The parameter estimate δ_q for the equate group is

$$\delta_q = \frac{\sum_{i \in Q} \delta_i w_i}{\sum_{i \in Q} w_i}$$

Equation 2.4.2.

2.4.5 COMMON LATENT SCALE

The end goal for using the equate group method to model development items is to measure development on one common latent scale, the D-score. That way, the measure (i.e. D-score) can be obtained, irrespective of which instrument is used in which population.

Figure 2.4.3 displays the D-score estimates by age in three cohorts from the GCDG study: Netherlands 1 (GCDG-NLS-SMOCC), Ethiopia (GCDG-ETH) and Colombia 2 (GCDG-COL-LT42M) for two different analyses. As described in section 2.2.2, the Netherlands 1 study administered the ddi; Ethiopia measured children by the by3; and Colombia collected data on by3, den, aqi and bdi. Accordingly, there is an overlap in items between Ethiopia and Colombia via the by3, but the Netherlands 1 cohort is not linked.

We created the plot on the left-hand side without active equate groups. The large overlap between Ethiopian and Columbian children occurs because the scales for these studies are linked naturally via shared items from by3. Since the ddi instrument is not connected, the Dutch cohort follows a different track. While we can compare D-scores between Ethiopia and Colombia, it is nonsensical to compare Dutch to either Ethiopia or Colombia. The right-hand side plot is based on an analysis that used active equate groups to link the cohorts. Since the analysis connected the scales for all three cohorts, we can now compare D-scores obtained between all three cohorts.

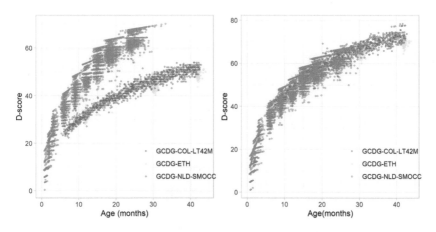

FIGURE 2.4.3 Example of three cohorts with and without equate group linking.

This example demonstrates that active equate groups form the key for converting ability estimates for children from different cohorts using different instruments onto the same scale.

2.4.6 QUANTIFYING EQUATE FIT

It is essential to activate only those equate groups for which the assumption of equivalent measurement holds. We have already seen the *item fit* and *person fit* diagnostics of the Rasch model. This section describes a similar measure for the quality of an active equate group.

2.4.6.1 EQUATE FIT

Section 1.6 defines the observed response of person n on item i as x_{ni}. The accompanying standardized residual z_{ni} is the difference between x_{ni} and the expected response P_{ni}, divided by the expected binomial standard deviation,

$$z_{ni} = \frac{x_{ni} - P_{ni}}{\sqrt{W_{ni}}}$$

with variances $W_{ni} = P_{ni}(1 - P_{ni})$.

Equate infit is an extension of item infit that takes an aggregate over all items i in active equate group q, i.e.,

$$\text{Equate infit} = \frac{\sum_{i \in q} \sum_{n}^{N} (x_{ni} - P_{ni})^2}{\sum_{i \in q} \sum_{n}^{N} W_{ni}}.$$

Likewise, we calculate *Equate outfit* of group q as

$$\textbf{Equate outfit} = \frac{\sum_{i \in q} \sum_n^{N_i} z_{ni}^2}{\sum_{i \in q} N_i},$$

where N_i is the total number of responses observed on item i. The interpretation of these diagnostics is the same as for item infit and item outfit.

Note that these definitions implicitly assume that the expected response P_{ni} is calculated under a model in which all items in equate group q have the same difficulty. This is not true for passive equate groups. Of course, no one can stop us from calculating the above equate fit statistics for passive groups, but such estimates would ignore the between-item variation in difficulties, and hence gives a too optimistic estimate of quality. The bottom line is: *The interpretation of the equate fit statistics should be restricted to active equate groups only.*

2.4.6.2   EXAMPLES OF WELL FITTING EQUATE GROUPS

The evaluation of *equate fit* involves comparing the observed probabilities of endorsing the items in the equate group to the estimated probability of endorsing the items in the equate group. For an equate group there is an empirical curve for each item in the equate group and one shared estimated curve. The empirical curves should all be close together, and close to the estimated curve for a good equate fit.

Figure 2.4.4 shows a diagnostic plot for equate groups REC6 (Turns head to sound of bell) and GM42 (Walks alone). The items within REC6 have slightly different formats in the Bayley I (by1), Dutch Development Instrument (ddi), and the Denver (den). The empirical curves in the upper figure show good overlap, but note that hardly any negative responses were recorded for four of the five studies, so the shared estimate depends primarily on the Dutch sample. Items from equate group GM42 appear in six instruments: bar, by1, by2, by3, ddi, and gri. Also, here the empirical data are close together, and even a little steeper than the fitted dashed line, which indicates a good equate fit. The infit and outfit indices, shown in the upper left corners, confirm the good fit (fit < 1).

2.4.6.3   EXAMPLES OF EQUATE GROUPS WITH POOR EQUATE FIT

Poor fitting equate groups are best treated as passive equate groups, so that items in those groups are not restricted to the same difficulty. Empirical item curves with different locations and slopes indicate a poor fit. Additionally, the equate fit indices will indicate a poor fit (fit > 1).

Figure 2.4.5 shows examples for groups COG24 (Bangs in play / Bangs 2 blocks) and EXP12 (Babbles). In both cases there is substantial variation in location between the empirical curves. For COG24 we find that the fitted curve

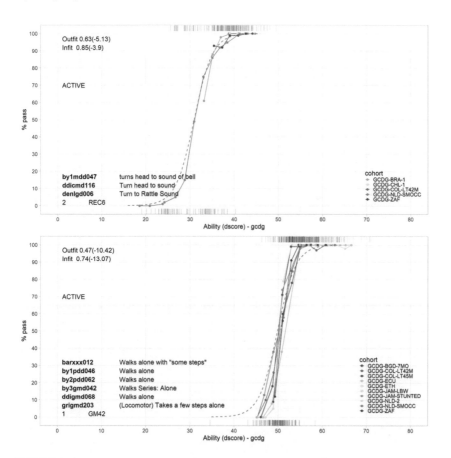

FIGURE 2.4.4   Two equate groups that present a good equate fit.

is closer to the `den` item, which suggests that the equate difficulty is mostly based on the `den` item. Items from equate group `EXP12` have a different format in instruments `by1`, `ddi` and `gri`. The empirical curves, with different colours for each instrument, are not close to each other, nor close to the fitted curve. Note that all infit and outfit statistics are fairly high, indicating poor fit. Both equates are candidates for deactivation in a next modelling step.

2.4.7   DIFFERENTIAL ITEM FUNCTIONING

Items within an active equate group should work in the same way across the different cohorts, i.e., they have no differential item functioning (DIF). The assumption of no DIF is critical for active equate groups. If violated, restricting the difficulty parameters as equal across cohorts may introduce unwanted bias in comparisons between cohorts. This section illustrates the role of DIF in equate groups.

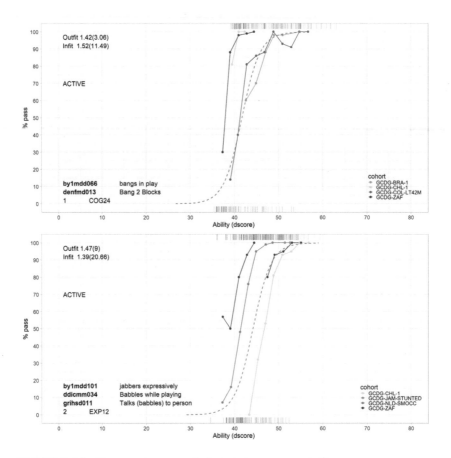

FIGURE 2.4.5   Two equate groups that present a poor equate fit.

2.4.7.1   GOOD EQUATE GROUPS WITHOUT **DIF**

Section 1.6.3 discusses the role of DIF in the evaluation of the fit of items to the Rasch model. This section illustrates similar issues in the context of equate groups.

Figure 2.4.6 shows the empirical curves of two equate groups, FM31 (two cubes) and EXP26 (two-word sentence). All curves are close to each other, so there is no differential item functioning here.

2.4.7.2   POOR EQUATE GROUPS WITH **DIF** FOR STUDY

Figure 2.4.7 plots the empirical curves for equate groups GM44 (throws ball) and EXP23 (5 or more words). The substantial variation between these curves

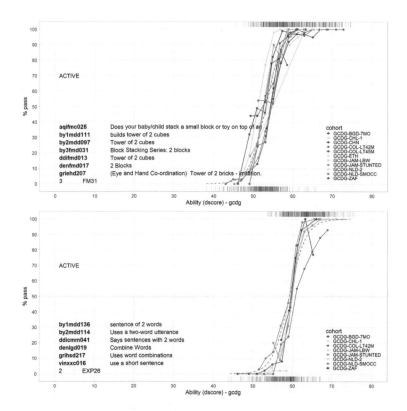

FIGURE 2.4.6 Two equate groups that present no differential item functioning between cohorts.

is a sign of differential item functioning. For example, *Throws ball* is easier for children in the South-Africa cohort (purple curve; GCDG-ZAF) and more difficult for children in Colombia (blue curve; GCDG-COL-LT42M). In other words, the probability of passing the item given the D-score (i.e. item difficulty) differs between the cohorts. Likewise, there is differential item functioning for *Says more than 5 words*. This milestone is easier for children in Jamaica (yellow and pink curves; GCDG-JAM-LBW and GCDG-JAM-STUNTED) than for children from Ecuador (green; GCDG-ECU).

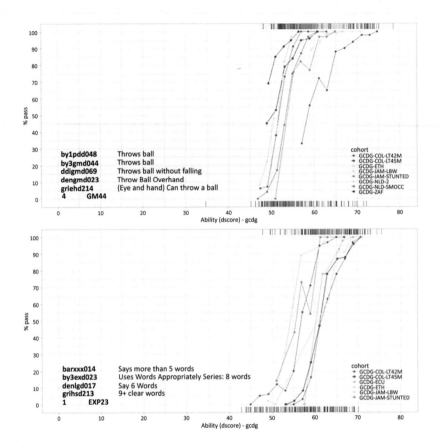

FIGURE 2.4.7 Two equate groups that present differential item functioning between cohorts.

2.5 Modelling equates

Iris Eekhout[1]
Stef van Buuren[1,2]
[1]Netherlands Organisation for Applied Scientific Research TNO, Leiden, 2316 ZL, The Netherlands
[2]University of Utrecht, Utrecht, 3584 CH, The Netherlands

This section deals with the nitty-gritty of the modelling strategy used for the GCDG data introduced in Section 2.2. This section

- provides a high-level description of the GCDG data (2.5.1)
- discusses various modelling strategies (2.5.2)
- shows the impact of equate groups on the model in extreme cases (2.5.3)
- demonstrates visualization of age profiles to select promising equate groups (2.5.4)
- introduces a helpful visualization of the quality of the equate group (2.5.5)
- highlights infit and outfit for removing misfitting milestones (2.5.6)
- discusses instrument fit and equate group editing (2.5.7)
- introduces a grading system for equate groups (2.5.8)
- provides pointers to the final model (2.5.9)

2.5.1 GCDG DATA: DESIGN AND DESCRIPTION

2.5.1.1 DATA COMBINATION

Section 2.2.1 provides an overview of the data collected by Global Child Development Group. The group collected item level measurements obtained on 12 instruments for measuring child development across 16 cohorts.

We coded every item as 0 (FAIL), 1 (PASS) or missing. For some instrument we did some additional recoding to restrict to these two response categories. The Battelle Developmental Inventory scores items as 0 (FAIL), 1, or 2, depending on the level of skill demonstrated or time taken to complete the task. We joined categories 1 and 2 for these items. The ASQ items were originally scored as 0 (not yet), 5 (sometimes) and 10 (succeeds). We recoded both 5 and 10 to 1.

We concatenated the datasets from the GCDG cohorts cohort. The resulting data matrix has 71403 rows (child-visit combinations) and 1572 columns (items) collected from 36345 unique children. We removed 233 items that had fewer than 10 observations in a category. The remaining 1339 items were candidates for analysis. The total number of observed scores was equal to about

2.8 million pass/fail responses. While this is a large number of measurements, about 97 percent of the entries in the matrix are missing.

2.5.1.2 Equate group formation

A group of 13 subject-matter experts from the Global Child Development Group cross-walked the available instruments for similar milestones. This group

- developed an item coding schema;
- matched similarly appearing items stemming from different instruments;
- formed an opinion about the quality of each match;
- noted peculiarities of the matches;
- reported the results as a series of detailed Excel spreadsheets.

The group evaluated around 1500 milestones. After several days, this highly-skilled, intensive labour resulted in a series of spreadsheets. Figure 2.5.1 shows an example. These sheets formed the basis of an initial list of 184 equate groups, each consisting of at least two items.

2.5.2 MODELLING STRATEGIES

The analytic challenge is twofold:

- to find a subset of items that form a scale;
- to find a subset of equate groups with items similar enough to bridge instruments.

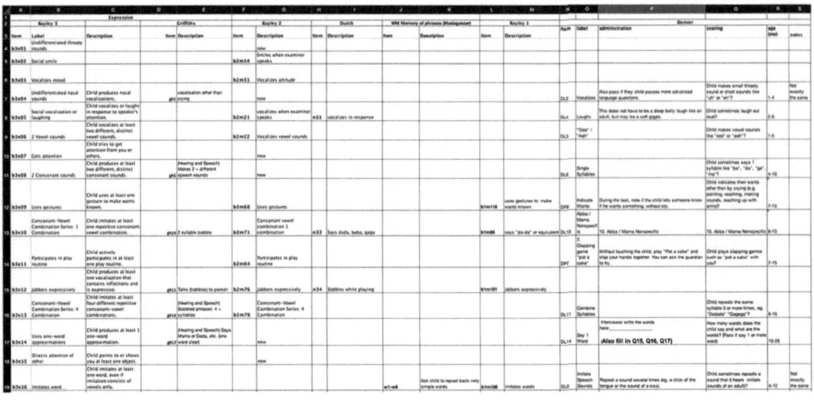

FIGURE 2.5.1 A snapshot of information generated by subject-matter experts.

Note that both subsets are related, i.e., changing one affects the other. Thus, we cannot first identify items and then equate groups, or first identify equate groups followed by the items. Rather we need to find the two subsets in an iterative fashion, primarily by hand. This section describes some of the modelling issues the analyst needs to confront.

In general, we look for a final model that

- preserves the items that best fit the Rasch model;
- uses active equate groups with items that behave the same across many cohorts and instruments;
- displays reasonable age-conditional distributions of the D-scores;
- has difficulty estimates that are similar to previous estimates.

The modelling strategy is a delicate balancing act to achieve all of the above objectives. Particular actions that we could take to improve a given model are:

- remove bad items;
- inactivate bad equate groups;
- break up bad equate groups;
- move items from one equate group to another;
- create new equate groups;
- remove entire instruments;
- remove persons;
- remove studies.

In order to steer our actions, we look at the following diagnostics (in order of importance):

- quality of equate groups (both visually and through infit);
- plausibility of the distribution of the D-score by age per study;
- correspondence of difficulty estimates from published (single study) Dutch data and the new model;
- infit of the items remaining in the model.

Various routes are possible and may result in different final models. The strategy adopted here is to thicken active equate groups by covering as many studies as possible, in the hope of minimizing the number of active equates needed.

2.5.3 IMPACT OF NUMBER OF ACTIVE EQUATE GROUPS

Figure 2.5.2 is a display of the D-score by age for the GCDG-COL-LT42M cohort under four models. D-score by age visualizations for all cohort are can be found via this link. As a rough reference to compare, the grey curves in the back represent the Dutch model as calculated from the SMOCC study. In order

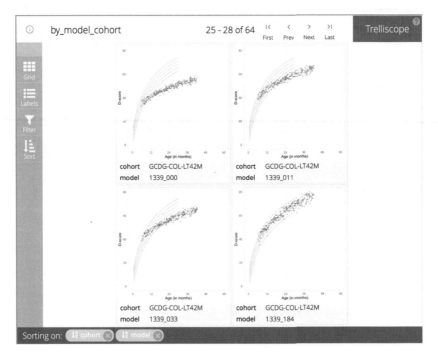

FIGURE 2.5.2 D-score by age of four models with all 1339 items using 0, 11, 33 and 184 active equate groups.

The number of equate groups has a substantial effect on the D-score distribution (https://d-score.org/dbook-apps/models1339/, in the online version you can use the arrows to see other cohorts).

to speed up the calculations, the figure shows a random subsample of 25% of all points. Manipulate the plot controls to switch cohorts.

All models contain 1339 items, but differ in the number of active equate groups. The most salient features per model are:

- 1339_: No equate groups, so different instruments in different cohorts are fitted independently;
- 1339_11: Connects all cohorts through one or more equated items using 11 equate groups in total;
- 1339_33: There are 33 equate groups that bridge cohort and instruments;
- 1339_184: Maximally connects instruments and cohort by all equate groups.

Comparison of the D-score distribution by age across these models yields various insights:

- The location of cohorts on the vertical scale depends on the number of active equate groups. For example, for Madagascar (MDG) the points are located around 52 when no equate groups are activated, whereas if all are activated it is about 68.
- The age trend depends on the number of active equate groups. For example, for Colombia (COL) or Ethiopia (ETH), the model without equate groups has a shallow age trend, whereas it is steep for the 1339_184 model.
- The vertical spread depends on the number of equate groups. For example, the spread in the Chile-2 (CHL-2) cohort substantially increases with the number of active equates.
- Model 1339_0 for the Dutch NLD-SMOCC cohort is equivalent to the model fitted to the SMOCC study alone. Introducing equate groups compresses the range of scores, especially at the higher end.

We have now seen that the number of active equate groups has a large effect on the model. The next sections look into the equate groups in more detail.

2.5.4 AGE PROFILES OF SIMILAR MILESTONES

Figure 2.5.3 displays the percentage of children that pass milestones at various ages for equate group EXP 26. Subject matter experts clustered similar items stemming from different instruments into equate groups. There are 184 equate groups that contain two or more milestones; the percentage pass by age for the items in these equate groups are shown here.

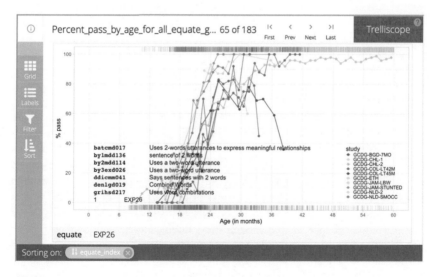

FIGURE 2.5.3 Percentage of children that pass similar milestones at a given age (https://d-score.org/dbook-apps/p-a-equate-1339/).

Most age profiles show a rising pattern, as expected, though some (e.g. FM17 or EXP11) have one item showing a negative relation with age. Equate EXP26 combines two-word sentences items from seven instruments into one plot. The item difficulties expressed as age-equivalents (cf. Section 1.3.1.2, Chapter I (van Buuren & Eekhout, 2021)) for these cohorts vary between 20–25 months. By comparison, equate group EXP18 (says two words) shows more heterogeneity across cohorts, and is therefore, less likely to be useful for equating. Equate group FM31 (stack two blocks) is another example of a promising example. By comparison, FM38 (stack 68 blocks) shows additional heterogeneity. As a last example, consider GM42 (walks alone), which has a similar age profile across cohorts, whereas GM44 (throws ball) or GM49 (walk down stairs) are more heterogeneous.

We could follow different strategies in selecting which equate groups to activate. One strategy would be to include as many equate groups as possible (e.g. all 184 equates) so as to build as many bridges as possible between different instruments. A more selective strategy would be to activate a subset of promising equates and leave others inactive. The following section compares four different approaches.

2.5.5 QUALITY OF EQUATE GROUPS

This visualization shows how the passing percentage depends on the child's D-score as calculated under four models. All models include the same 1339 milestones, but differ in the number of active equates. The grey curve corresponds to the estimate made under the assumption that milestones are equally difficult. Good milestones for bridging instruments will have a tight bundle of curves. For example, as shown in Figure 2.5.4, equate EXP26 has tight bundles especially in models 1339_11 and 1339_33. By comparison, the curves of the two extreme models vary considerably: the model without any bridges (1339_) or the model with all bridges (1339_184) are thus less than ideal. The shallow grey curve of model 1339_184 indicates a poorer overall fit.

Outfit and infit statistics measure the residual deviation of the items to the grey curve. High values (e.g. above 1.4) are undesirable and indicate lack of fit to the model. For example, the fit statistics for EXP26 in model 1339_184 (1.70 and 1.25) indicate a mediocre fit, whereas EXP26 in models 1339_33 and 1339_11 fits well. Sometimes the individual item curves are steeper than the grey curve. This indicates that these milestones are more discriminative than the combined item. Model 1339_ lacks a grey curve and has no fit statistics for equate groups, because in that model, the combined item is not activated.

The probability curves provide a quick visual method for spotting promising and problematic equate groups. Examples of promising equate groups include COG36, FM31, GM26 and GM42. A little more weak are FM26 (has more variability), FM52 (looks promising, but has a problem with the item grigcd42 from the GCDG_JAM_STUNTED cohort), and GM35 (does not align cohort

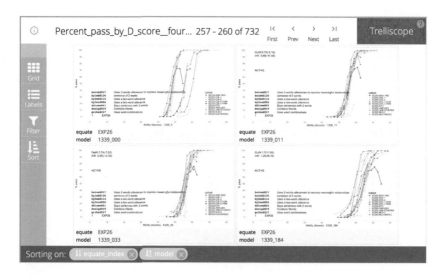

FIGURE 2.5.4   Percentage of children that pass similar milestones given their D-score as calculated under four models (1339 items, and 0, 11, 33 and 184 equate groups, respectively (https://d-score.org/dbook-apps/p-d-equate-1339/).

GCDG-ZAF). In such cases, one may wish to move an item out of an equate group, combine equate groups, or inactivate troublesome links.

Until now we only looked at models that include all 1339 items. In practice, we may improve upon the model by selecting the subset of milestones that fit the Rasch model. The next section looks in this modelling step in more detail.

2.5.6   MILESTONE SELECTION

Item infit and outfit are convenient statistics for selecting the milestones that fit the model. Figure 2.5.5 displays the infit and outfit statistics of model 1339_11. The correlation between infit and outfit is high ($r = 0.84$). The expected value of the infit and outfit statistics for a perfect fit is 1.0. The centre of infit and outfit in Figure 2.5.5 is approximately 1.0, so on average one could say the items fit the model. Note however that fit values above and below the values of 1.0 are qualitatively different. Item with fit statistics exceeding 1.0 fit the model less well than expected (**underfit**), whereas items with fit statistics lower than 1.0 fit the model better than expected (**overfit**). See Chapter 1, Section 6.1 (van Buuren & Eekhout, 2021) for more details.

Some practitioners remove both underfitting and overfitting items. However, we like to preserve overfitting items and be more strict in removing items that underfit. The idea is that preservation of the best fitting items may increase scale length, and hence reliability and measurement precision. Figure 2.5.5 draws two cut-off lines at 1.0. Taking items with infit < 1.0 and outfit < 1.0 will select **631 out of 1339** items for further modelling.

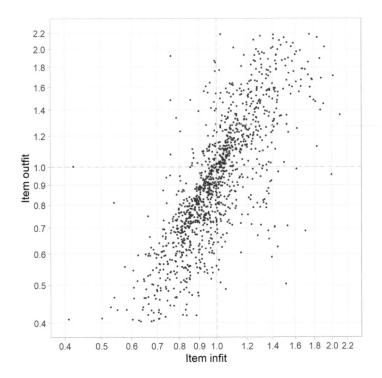

FIGURE 2.5.5   Infit and outfit of 1339 items in model `1339_11`.

About 8 percent of the points falls outside the plot.

A practical problem of item removal is that it also affects equate group composition. By default, a removed item will also be removed from the equate group, so item removal may reduce the size of an equate group below two items. For passive equates this is no problem, since passive equates do no affect the estimates. However, removal of an underfitting item from an active equate group will break the bridge between the instrument it pertains to and the rest of the item set. Potentially this can result in substantial effects on the D-score distribution of the cohort, as demonstrated in Figure 2.5.2. As a solution, we force any items that are members of active equate groups to remain in the analysis. If that leads to substantially worse equate fit in the next model, we must search for alternative equate groups that bridge the same instruments and that are less sensitive to misfit.

2.5.7   OTHER MODELLING ACTIONS

2.5.7.1   INSTRUMENT FIT

Some instruments fit better than others. Figure 2.5.6 shows the box plots of outfit per instrument. Instruments `bar`, `by1`, `ddi` and `vin` generally fit well,

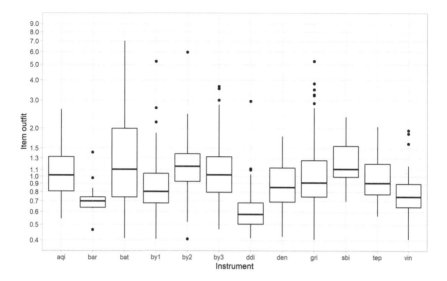

FIGURE 2.5.6 Box plot of the distribution of item outfit per instrument in model 1339_11.

whereas discrepancies between model and data are larger for bat, by2 and sbi. Through additional modelling, we found that it was extremely difficult to get enough high-quality bridge items that could link bat (Battelle Development Inventory) to the other instruments. We also found that models without the Battelle were able to better discriminate children in the upper range of the D-score scale. We therefore opted to remove bat from the model, even though this meant that one cohort (GCDG-BRA-2) had to be dropped from the analysis.

It is not clear why bat does not fit. Perhaps the scoring system of the Battelle in three categories invokes scoring behaviour that is different from the PASS/ FAIL scoring used by most other instruments, even though this appears to be less of a troublesome aspect in aqi, which also uses three response categories.

2.5.7.2 SPLITTING, COMBINING AND SELECTING EQUATE GROUPS

Most of the modelling effort went into finding a set of high-quality equate groups that link the instruments. For example, we tried to bridge the South-African study placing vinxxc016 (uses a short sentence) into EXP26 (two-word sentences) and EXP36 (sentences of 3 or more words), but neither option led to a reasonable model. On the surface, milestone reasonable model. On the surface, milestone by3gmd06 (balances on right foot, 2 seconds) appears to fit within GM60 (balances on foot), but the analysis showed large discrepancies with the other items in the groups, so it had to be taken out.

Subject-matter experts identified 38 items that were thought to be cross-culturally incompatible. Table 2.5.1 provides an overview. Many of such milestones involve a specific language concept (such as a pronoun), refer to stairs (less common

TABLE 2.5.1

Milestones not used for equating because of limited cross-cultural validity.

Item	Label
aqislc023	When you dress your baby does she lift her foot for her shoe, sock, or pant leg?
aqislc041	Using these exact words, ask your child, "Are you a girl or a boy?" Does your child answer correctly?
by1mdd050	Washes and dries hands
by1pdd053	Bowel and bladder control
by1pdd054	manipulates table edge actively
by2pdd069	Walsk up stairs with help
by3cgd043	Walks down stairs with help
by3cgd052	Walks down stairs with help
by3gmd047	Clear Box: Front
by3gmd049	Clear Box: Sides
by3gmd057	Uses pronouns
by3gmd058	Walks Up Stairs Series: Both feet on each step, with support.
by3red030	Walks Down Stairs Series: Both feet on each step, with support
by3exd030	Walks Up Stairs Series: Both feet on each step, alone.
barxxx016	Walks Down Stairs Series: Both feet on each step, alone
barxxx020	Understands pronouns (him, me, my, you, your)
dengmd020	Eats with spoon without help (M; can ask parents)
densld012	Takes off shoes and socks (M; can ask parents)
densld013	Can dress (one piece) (M; can ask parents)
grigmd219	Walk Up Stairs
grigmd222	Drink from a cup
mdsgmd002	help in house
mdsgmd003	(Locomotor) Walks up and down stairs.
mdsgmd004	(Locomotor) Goes alone on the stairs (any method)
mdsgmd005	Hands-and-knees crawling
mdsgmd006	Standing with assistance
ddifmm019	Walking with assistance
ddifmd154	Standing alone
vinxxc002	Walking alone
vinxxc003	chew solid foods
vinxxc009	take off socks / shoes
vinxxc012	get on with other children
vinxxc014	know what's edible
vinxxc022	walk upstairs
vinxxc028	avoid simple danger - knife / hot
vinxxc031	help around the house / clear table
vinxxc040	Play or do things with other children of same age eg sing song
ddifmm025	Help with little things around the house eg pick up things

in rural settings), help in house or clothing behaviour. These items have different meanings in different contexts, so they were not used to bridge instruments.

2.5.8   ITEM INFORMATION

Item information is a psychometric measure that quantifies the sensitivity of the item to changes in the person's ability. An item is most sensitive around the D-score value where the PASS probability equals the FAIL probability, which corresponds to the item difficulty (δ_i). One unit change around δ_i has a large effect on the probability of endorsing, while one unit change far away from δ_i has negligible impact. Suppose person A had passing probability 0.7 for some item. The information delivered by that item for person A is the product $0.7 \times (1.0 - 0.7) = 0.21$. Suppose person B has a D-score that coincides with the difficulty level of the item. In that case, the information for B equals $0.5 \times (1 - 0.5) = 0.25$, the maximum. Likewise, for a person C with high ability, the information could be $0.98 \times 0.02 = 0.02$, so that item carries almost no information for person C.

The information is inversely related to the error of measurement. More information amounts to less measurement error. For each response in the data, we can compute the amount of information it contributed to the model D-score. By summing the information over persons, we obtain a measure of certainty about the difficulty estimate of the item. This sum of information incorporates both the number of administrations and the quality of the match between person abilities and item difficulty.

Figure 2.5.7 displays the summed information for each item, divided into four grades: A(best) to D (worst). The information grade measures the stability of the difficulty estimate. Most items receive grades higher than C. In total, 30 milestones have grade D. Adding these items to future studies may yield important additional information.

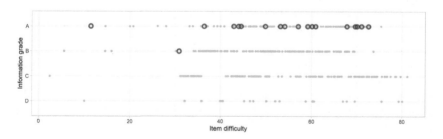

FIGURE 2.5.7   Item information grade by item difficulty for the final model.

TABLE 2.5.2
Equate group information in the final model.

equate	tau	n	info	grade
EXP2	11.44	3608	162.33	A
REC6	30.9	5428	95.40	B
GM25	36.43	6380	470.63	A
FM26	42.93	4155	296.78	A
GM35	44.01	5522	356.04	A
COG36	44.53	7912	230.03	A
GM42	49.86	5953	327.74	A
FM31	53.17	10991	731.66	A
COG55	54.08	5647	420.35	A
FM72	57.07	5430	253.64	A
EXP26	59.15	9119	578.79	A
SA1	60.08	3363	172.11	A
FM38	60.87	10236	491.68	A
FM52	67.8	13487	1159.94	A
FM43	69.66	15765	1563.89	A
GM60	70.09	9519	1070.61	A
REC40	71.04	10393	1182.91	A
FM61	72.56	10612	945.87	A

The red circles indicate active equate groups. Most have grade A, so we have a lot of information about the items that form the active equate groups. Table 2.5.2 displays more detailed information for the active equate groups. The sample sizes are reasonably large. Many information statistics are well is above 100; the criterion for Grade A. The interpretation of this criterion is as follows. Suppose that we obtain a sample of 400 persons who are all perfectly calibrated to the item of interest. In that case, the information for that item will be equal to 100.

2.5.9   FINAL MODEL

Unfortunately, there is no single index of model fit that we can optimize. Modelling is more like a balancing act among multiple competing objectives, such as

- preserving as many items as possible that fit the model;
- finding high-quality active equate groups that span many cohorts and instruments;
- picking active equate groups for which we have enough information;
- providing reasonable age-conditional distributions of the D-score;

- representing various developmental domains in a fair way;
- preserving well-fitting historical models as new data become available;
- maintaining a reasonable calculation time.

This section showed various modelling techniques and ways to assess the validity of the model. In real life, we fitted a total number of 140 models on the data and made many choices that weigh the above objectives. The final model for the GCDG data consists of 565 items (originating from 14 instruments) that fit the Rasch model and that connect through 18 equate groups. Due to the sparseness of data at the very young ages, the quality of the model is best for ages between 4–36 months.

Model 565_18 formed the basis of the publication by Weber *et al.* (2019). Additional detail on model 565_18 is available through the dmodel shiny app at https://tnochildhealthstatistics.shinyapps.io/dmodel/.

2.6 Comparing ability

Iris Eekhout[1]
Stef van Buuren[1,2]
[1]Netherlands Organisation for Applied Scientific Research TNO, Leiden, 2316 ZL, The Netherlands
[2]University of Utrecht, Utrecht, 3584 CH, The Netherlands

Once we identified a satisfactory D-score model, we may calculate the D-score for children from different cohorts and compare their values. This section highlights various techniques and issues for comparing D-score distributions between studies. We will address the following topics:

- Comparing child development across studies (2.6.1)
- Precision of the D-score (2.6.2)
- Domain coverage (2.6.3)

2.6.1 COMPARING CHILD DEVELOPMENT ACROSS STUDIES

This display shows the scatterplot of the D-score by age separately for each cohort, Figure 2.6.1 presents the D-score by age for the GCDG-COL-LT52M study. Remember from section 2.2.1 that each study selected its own set of instruments to collect the data. The scatterplots demonstrate a significant advance made possible by the D-score: We can plot the developmental scores of children from **different** cohorts, with **different** ages, using **different** instruments, on the **same** vertical axis.

The five blue lines guide the eye. These lines indicate the locations of the -2SD, -1SD, 0SD, +1SD and +2SD quantiles at each age in the combined data. Section 2.5.4, in Chapter I (van Buuren & Eekhout, 2021) motivates the idea and provides some technical details. We'll come back to these lines in section 2.7.2.

By and large, the data in every study follow the blue lines. Perhaps the most obvious exception is the GCDG-JAM-STUNTED cohort, where older children somewhat exceed the D-score range. It is unknown whether this is real, or due to a sub-optimal calibration of the instrument.

Figure 2.6.2 plots the same data with D-score transformed into age standardized scores (DAZ) for study GCDG-COL-LT42M. The distributions of the age standardized scores for all studies are displayed here. Replacing the D-score by the DAZ emphasizes the differences both within and between studies. The majority of observations lies between the -2 SD and +2 SD lines in all cohorts. Using DAZ makes is easier to spot deviating trends, e.g., for the Jamaican or Ethiopian data.

DOI: 10.1201/9781003216315-17

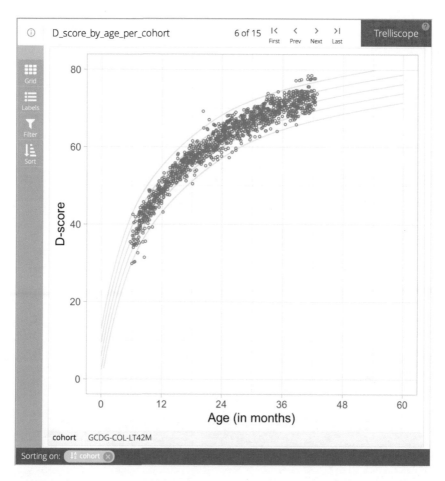

FIGURE 2.6.1 D-score distributions for study GCDG-COL-LT42M (https://d-score. org/dbook-apps/gcdgdscores/).

2.6.2 PRECISION OF THE D-SCORE

The EAP algorithm estimates the D-score from a set of PASS/FAIL scores. The standard deviation of the posterior distribution (or *sem*: standard error of measurement) quantifies the imprecision of the D-score estimate. The *sem* is inversely related to the number of items. Thus, when we administer more milestones, the *sem* of the D-score drops.

Figure 2.6.3 shows that the *sem* drops off rapidly when the number of items is low and stabilizes after about 35 items. Apart from test length, the precision of the D-score also depends on item information (cf. section 2.5.8). Administering items that are too easy, or too difficult, does not improve precision. The figure suggests that - in practice - a single D-score cannot be more precise than 0.5 D-score units.

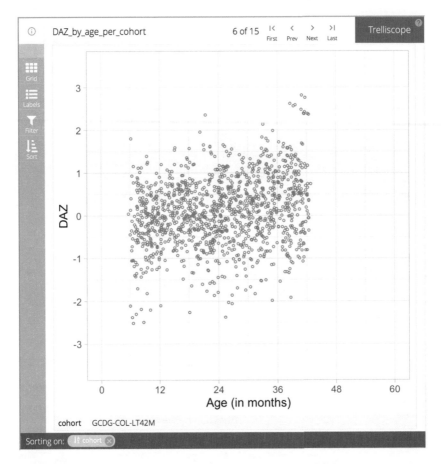

FIGURE 2.6.2 DAZ distributions for study GCDG-COL-LT42M (https://d-score.org/dbook-apps/gcdgdaz/).

One may wonder whether the *sem* depends on age. Figure 2.6.4 suggests that this is not the case. The average DAZ is close to zero everywhere, as expected. The interval DAZ ± *sem* will cover the true, but unknown, DAZ in about 68% of the cases. While the interval varies somewhat across ages, there is no systematic age trend.

Does precision vary with studies? The answer is yes. Figure 2.6.5 plots the same information as before but now only for GCDG-COL-LT42M. The standard error of measurement around de age-standardized D-scores (DAZ) for each cohort can be found here. Individual data points are added to give a feel for the design. The Colombia cohort GCDG-COL-LT45M, Figure 2.6.5, administered the Bayley-III, where each child answered on average 45 items, so the *sem* is small. In contrast, the Dutch cohort GCDG-NLD-SMOCC collected data on a screener consisting of about ten relatively easy milestones, so the *sem*

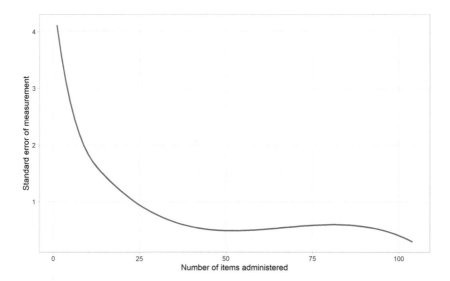

FIGURE 2.6.3 Standard error of measurement (sem) as a function of the number of items.

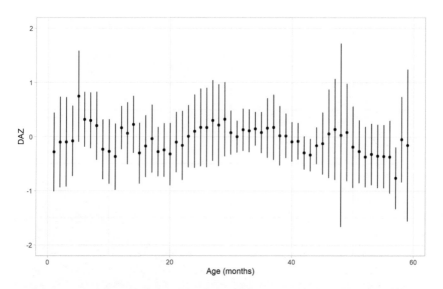

FIGURE 2.6.4 Mean DAZ ± sem as a function of age.

is relatively large. As a result, the Colombian D-scores are much more precise than the Dutch. These differences in precision between cohorts is also reflected in Figure 2.6.6. This figure shows the pooled standard error of measurement within each cohort.

The ordering of studies depends on test length and item information. Table 2.6.1 shows the median number of items per child (test length) and the

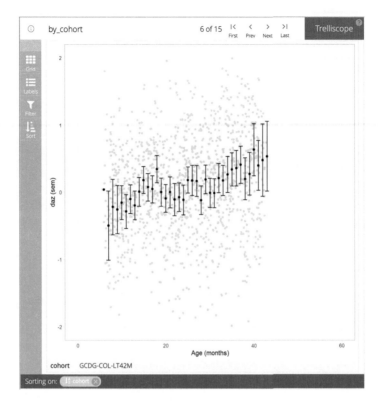

FIGURE 2.6.5   The standard error of measurement (sem) around the age-standardized D-scores (DAZ) for cohort **GCDG-COL-LT42M** (https://d-score.org/dbook-apps/gcdgsem).

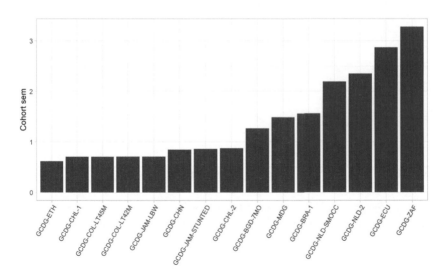

FIGURE 2.6.6   Cohort Standard Error of Measurement (sem).

TABLE 2.6.1
Test length and probability to pass the items per cohort.

cohort	test length (median)	pass probability (median)
GCDG-ETH	39	0,66
GCDG-CHL-1	32	0,67
GCDG-COL-LT45M	45	0,64
GCDG-COL-LT42M	61	0,62
GCDG-JAM-LBW	43	0,55
GCDG-CHN	27	0,50
GCDG-JAM-STUNTED	38	0,65
GCDG-CHL-2	33	0,48
GCDG-BGD-7MO	14	0,38
GCDG-MDG	8	0,35
GCDG-BRA-1	18	0,89
GCDG-NLD-SMOCC	10	0,80
GCDG-NLD-2	11	1,00
GCDG-ECU	3	0,67
GCDG-ZAF	12	1,00

probability to pass the item. The Ethiopian cohort GCDG-ETH administered 39 milestones with a median probability of 0.66. In contrast, the South Africa study GCDG-ZAF measures 12 items which were all very easy for the sample at hand (median probability of 1.0). One may thus well explain the extremes by test length and item information.

In general, the design of the study has a significant impact on the precision of the measurement. Our ongoing work addresses the question how one may construct a measurement instrument that will be optimally precise given the goals of the research.

2.6.3 DOMAIN COVERAGE

The D-score is a one-number summary of early child development. Traditional instruments distinguish domains (like motor, communication, language and cognitive development) and some provide ways to calculate a total score. The D-score, on the other hand, is based on the notion that child development is a unidimensional latent construct and hence does not provide domain scores. And thus, the question is how the D-score represents domains.

This section explores the following two questions:

- Can we break down the D-score by domain contribution, and if so, can we evaluate whether the D-score fairly represents all domains?
- Can we calculate domain-specific D-scores?

2.6.3.1 DOMAIN COVERAGE OF THE SCALE

For many items in the D-score model, we had expert information available as to which domain the item belongs. For each item, we calculated the proportion of times the experts assigned it to one of five domains: Fine Motor, Gross Motor, Expressive, Receptive, Cognitive. We then calculated the distribution of domain by age.

Figure 2.6.7 shows the domain composition of the D-score across different levels of ability. Note that we miss domain information for a few items. The share of gross-motor is large in early development (e.g., between 15 and 30 months), and gradually tapers off at higher levels. Reversely, the percentage of cognition and language is relatively small before 30 months but rapidly rises as the child matures. These transitions in domain composition look both reasonable and valid.

2.6.3.2 DOMAIN-SPECIFIC D-SCORES

Suppose we select a domain of interest and calculate the D-score only from items that substantially load onto that domain. We then get a domain-specific D-score. Items that relate to multiple domains contribute to multiple domain-specific D-scores.

Figure 2.6.8 displays the standardized domain-specific D-score (i.e. DAZ) per cohort. The DAZ strips out irrelevant age variation, and thus enhances comparability between cohorts. The error bars around the scores depict the *sem* interval. We observe some variation in domain-specific DAZ scores within cohorts. Still, these differences are relatively small and well within the margins of error. This analysis suggests that the D-score is an excellent overall summary of the domain-specific D-scores.

The D-score methodology assumes that child development is a unidimensional scale. As a consequence, the correlations between different domain-specific

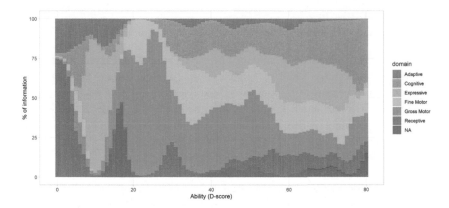

FIGURE 2.6.7   Domain coverage of the D-score scale.

D-scores are extremely high ($r > 0.95$). It is more interesting to study the correlation between the DAZ equivalent of the domain-specific scores.

Table 2.6.2 lists the Pearson correlation matrix of the DAZ and the five domain-specific DAZ scores. All correlations between the DAZ and the domain-specific scores are high, thus confirming the generic character of the D-score and DAZ. We find high inter-domain correlations for the cognitive-receptive, cognitive-fine motor and expressive-receptive pairs. The gross motor domain appears as somewhat distinct from the four other domains. Its position may be genuine, but could also be related to the smaller number of responses on gross motor milestones in the GCDG data.

Figure 2.6.9 displays individual scores for a 3 year old boy. The filled bars indicate the number of available items per domain. The vertical white line that crosses the horizontal axis at value 5 indicates a threshold for a minimum number of items needed for a D-score. Note that the number of items for Gross Motor in this example is meagre (only three items). The grey vertical line indicates the value of the overall D-score (68.55 D). The nearby dashed lines are located at one *sem* (0.53 D) distance. The coloured points are the domain-

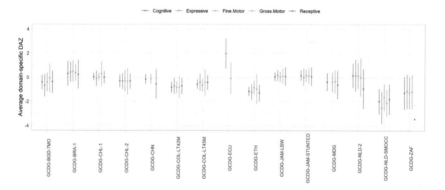

FIGURE 2.6.8 Average domain-specific DAZ ± sem by cohort.

TABLE 2.6.2

Pearson correlation of the DAZ and five domain-specific DAZ scores.

	DAZ	Fine motor	Gross Motor	Cognitive	Receptive	Expressive
DAZ	1.00	0.69	0.57	0.84	0.70	0.69
Fine motor	0.69	1.00	0.40	0.74	0.50	0.39
Gross Motor	0.57	0.40	1.00	0.43	0.34	0.30
Cognitive	0.84	0.74	0.43	1.00	0.76	0.59
Receptive	0.70	0.50	0.34	0.76	1.00	0.63
Expressive	0.69	0.39	0.30	0.59	0.63	1.00

specific D-scores with the *sem* around in error bars. The plot visualizes that the boys' scores on language domains (i.e. Expressive and Receptive) are low as compared to the motor and cognitive domains. A systematic discrepancy between various domain-specific scores might be an early warning sign for developmental delay.

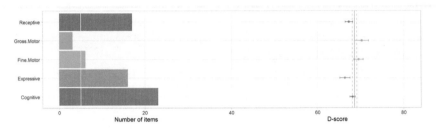

FIGURE 2.6.9   Domain-specific D-scores for a 3 year old boy.

2.7 Application I: tracking a Sustainable Development Goal

Iris Eekhout[1]
Stef van Buuren[1,2]
[1]Netherlands Organisation for Applied Scientific Research TNO, Leiden, 2316 ZL, The Netherlands
[2]University of Utrecht, Utrecht, 3584 CH, The Netherlands

The Sustainable Development Goals (SDG) formulated by the United Nations (UN) set targets to promote prosperity while protecting the planet. One or more indicators quantify the progress towards each target.

This section explores the use of the D-score to monitor the progress of the indicator for healthy child development, SDG 4.2.1. We propose a method to define on-track development and show how the application of this method pans out for the GCDG data. More in detail, the section deals with the following topics:

- Estimating SDG 4.2.1 indicator from existing data (2.7.1)
- Defining *developmentally on track* (2.7.2)
- Country-level estimations (2.7.3)
- Relation to other estimates (2.7.4)

2.7.1 ESTIMATING SDG 4.2.1 INDICATOR FROM EXISTING DATA

The UN Sustainable Development Goals form a universal call to action to end poverty, protect the planet and improve the lives and prospects of everyone, everywhere. All UN Member States adopted the 17 Goals in 2015. The SDG 4 target to ensure inclusive and equitable quality education and promote lifelong learning opportunities for all. SDG 4.2 reads as:

> By 2030, ensure that all girls and boys have access to quality early childhood development, care and preprimary education so that they are ready for primary education.

DOI: 10.1201/9781003216315-18

To measure progress, the UN defined indicator 4.2.1 as follows:

Proportion of children under 5 years of age who are developmentally on track in health, learning and psychosocial well-being, by sex.

On July 22, 2020, the indicator was changed into

Proportion of children aged 24–59 months who are developmentally on track in health, learning and psychosocial well-being, by sex.

The exclusion of children 0–24 months is at variance with the importance of healthy growth and development during the first 1000 days of life. Indeed, the UN restricted the age range for practical concerns. Loizillon *et al.* (2017) report:

The initial recommendation was for the ECDI to measure child development from birth–5 years, but the range was restricted to 3–5 years due to time and resource constraints and limited availability of comparable measurement tools for children under age 3.

The careful scientific approach underlying the D-score fills the gap for children aged 0–24 months. Also, the D-score methodology enables extensions to ages beyond 24 months, permits back-calculation of D-scores from existing data, and acts as a linking pin to compare child development from birth onwards.

The cohorts included in the GCDG study represent a wide range of countries and instruments (see Section 2.2.1). Combining existing data from such a wide range of countries to create the D-score, is undoubtedly challenging, but doable. Although, in all fairness, we note that obtaining accurate comparisons between world-wide populations requires additional representative (existing) data beyond what is available here.

2.7.2   DEFINING DEVELOPMENTALLY ON TRACK

In 2006, the World Health Organization (WHO) published the WHO Child Growth Standards. These standards specify "how children should grow" and form the basis for widely used anthropometric indicators such as stunting and wasting. We advocate a similar approach for child development. More in particular, the following steps:

1. Measure child development on an interval scale;
2. Estimate the age-conditional reference distribution for normal child development;
3. Define the indicator *developmentally on track* as the proportion above a chosen cut-off.

Step 1 is solved by the D-score. Step 2 borrows from well-tested statistical methodology for constructing growth standards (Borghi *et al.*, 2006). Step 3 can be done in different ways, but a applying a simple cut-off fits easily with regular practice in reporting international comparisons.

Figure 2.7.1 demonstrates steps 2 and 3 in more detail. In the online visualization you can click "Next" to advance these series of six steps:

1. Plot the D-score by age;
2. Model the relation between age and D-score by an LMS model. In practice, this amounts to smoothing three curves representing the median, coefficient of variation and the skewness.
3. Present the centile lines for the model;
4. Plot the age-standardized scores for development (DAZ);
5. Draw standard deviation lines to indicate the location at ±1 and ±2 standard deviation from the mean;
6. Count observations above the -2 SD line as on-track. Count observation below the -2 SD lines as off-track (red dots).

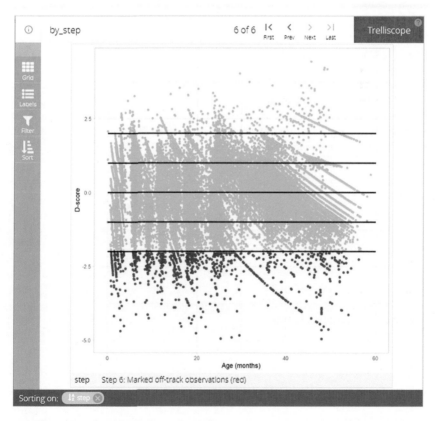

FIGURE 2.7.1 Illustration of the method to define on-track development (https:// d-score.org/dbook-apps/gcdgreferences/).

Note: The SD lines as presented in Figure 2.7.1, are built upon on a convenience sample. The GCDG cohorts are not representative samples, and the countries are not representative of the world. While we should not over-interpret these references, they play a central role in a stepwise, principled approach to define "developmentally on track."

2.7.3   COUNTRY-LEVEL ESTIMATIONS

Using the definition from the previous section, we can calculate the percentage of children that are developmentally on track. Table 2.7.1 summarizes this statistic by country. At a cut-off value of -2 SD, we expect that about 97.7% of the children will be on track. The actual country estimates fall into the range 93.9 - 99.9 and are thus near the theoretical value. This close correspondence shows that the definition and estimation procedure work as expected.

Bear in mind that the measurements leading up to these estimates come from different instruments. It is gratifying to see how well we can do with historical data, thanks to the robust underlying measurement model. Of course, comparability only gets better if all countries would use the same instrument. However, using the same tool everywhere is not a requirement.

2.7.4   OFF-TRACK DEVELOPMENT AND STUNTED GROWTH

Weber *et al.* (2019) thoroughly discuss concurrent, discriminant and predictive validity of the D-score using the GCDG data. In this section, we concentrate on the relation between the D-score and stunting, a popular measure of impaired height growth in children due to nutrition problems. The WHO defines stunted growth as a height-for-age Z-score below the -2 SD line of the WHO Child Growth Standards (HAZ < -2.0).

TABLE 2.7.1

Percentage of on-track children per country.

Country	Percentage on-track
BGD	94.9
BRA	99.5
CHL	98.3
CHN	99.9
COL	98.8
ECU	93.9
ETH	99.4
JAM	99.6
MDG	96.6
NLD	96.8
ZAF	97.4

Figure 2.7.2 plots the percentage off-track and percentage stunting per country. This plot reveals two exciting features:

- *The variation in stunting is much larger than the variation off-track development.* One might speculate that height is more dependent on the environment than off-track development, and hence more variable.
- *Stunted growth and off-track development are unrelated.* Ranking countries by stunting or by off-track development yields substantially different orders. This finding provides clear counter-evidence to the argument that stunted growth is as a proxy for delayed development. It may even be the case the child development and physical growth are different maturation processes that develop largely independently.

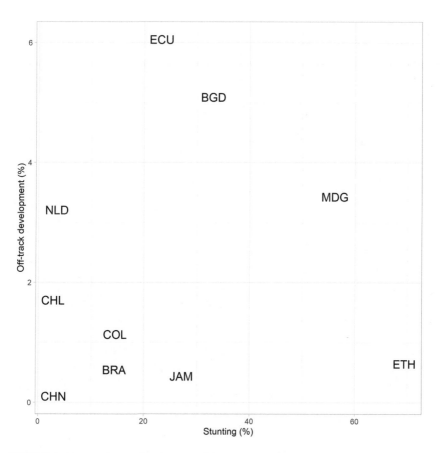

FIGURE 2.7.2 Off-track development (%) versus stunting (%) per country.

However, this is not the whole story. Figure 2.7.3 reveals a consistent difference in DAZ between stunted and non-stunted children of about 0.2-0.3 SD. There could be factors at the child level that affect both development and height growth. For example, low-income families may lack the resources for adequate nutrition, which may impact both child development and physical growth.

The exact nature of the relation between stunting and development is still obscure. The D-score provides a means to study the intriguing interplay between both measures in more detail.

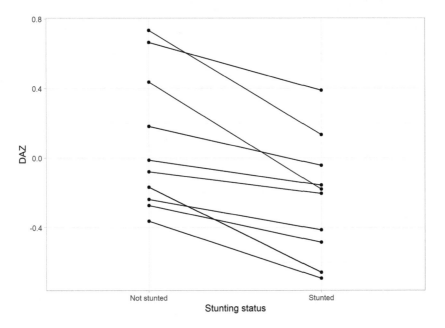

FIGURE 2.7.3   Difference in mean DAZ per country between stunted and not stunted children.

2.8 Application II: who is on-track?

Iris Eekhout[1]
Stef van Buuren[1,2]
[1]Netherlands Organisation for Applied Scientific Research TNO, Leiden, 2316 ZL, The Netherlands
[2]University of Utrecht, Utrecht, 3584 CH, The Netherlands

Section 2.7 described a method to define and estimate off-track development. The current section highlights strategies to find factors that discriminate between children that are on-track and off-track. We order explanatory factors relative to their importance and discuss opportunities for interventions.

- What determines who is developmentally on-track (2.8.1)
- Factors that impact child development (2.8.2)

2.8.1 WHAT DETERMINES WHO IS DEVELOPMENTALLY ON-TRACK?

There are multiple ways to define on-track development. Here we will use the method outlined in Section 2.7.2. Ideally, we would like to fit the age-conditional reference distribution on a sample of children with normal, healthy development. As noted before, we calculated the references used in Section 2.7.2 from a convenience sample. They may not be representative of healthy development.

Assuming we place the cut-off value at -2 SD, we may subdivide the observed D-scores into off-track and on-track. Figure 2.8.1 colours the regions of the D-score for children considered on-track (green) and off-track (red). The regions indicate the expected locations of D-scores in practice. Although one could find D-score outside the coloured areas, such should be very rare. The occurrence of such cases may indicate an error in the calculation of the D-score, most likely caused by setting an incorrect age variable.

Preventing observations in the red region requires us to form an idea about the factors that determine the off-track probability. The next section looks into this topic.

2.8.2 FACTORS THAT IMPACT CHILD DEVELOPMENT

We already know many of the factors that influence early child development. A higher level of education in the family promotes development. Infectious

DOI: 10.1201/9781003216315-19

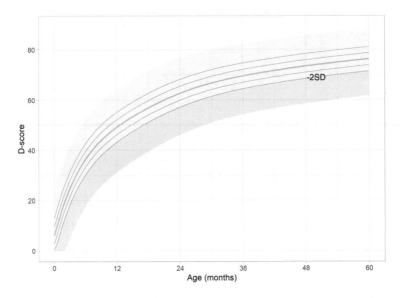

FIGURE 2.8.1   D-score observatations that are on-track according the current references.

diseases like malaria slow down growth. Access to adequate nutrition, clean water and a stimulating, prosperous and safe environment is favourable for healthy development. And so on. Unfortunately, we do not have data on most factors, so we need to limit ourselves to a few background characteristics.

Table 2.8.1 compares the frequency distributions of various factors for children on-track versus off-track. There are only tiny differences between boys and girls. Children with low birth weight (< 2500 gr) are more at risk for off-track development. This estimate does not correct for gestational age. We discussed techniques for such corrections elsewhere.

The influence of maternal education on off-track development follows the expected trend. Interestingly, it seems that a rural environment could prevent off-track development. We note that original measures of maternal education and residence were harmonized across studies. It would, therefore, also be interesting to study the impact per cohort using the actual factor coding.

We predicted DAZ by linear regressions with predictors country, sex, birth weight, maternal education, height for age and residential area. The percentage of explained variance was 11 percent. Figure 2.8.2 depicts the relative contributions of the individual factors to the prediction. Country differences explain over half the variances, followed by maternal education. Contributions of height-for-age (HAZ), low birth weight and residence are about equal in magnitude.

These analyses only scratch the surface. It is nowadays common to analyse the impact of interventions on height and HAZ by multivariate techniques and machine learning methods. The D-score and DAZ are drop-in replacements that allow similar procedures to study which factors contribute to healthy child development worldwide.

TABLE 2.8.1
Comparisons between on-track and off-track development.

		On-track		Off-track	
		n	%	n	%
sex	female	21136	97.7	489	2.3
	male	20805	97.2	595	2.8
birth weight	<2500gr	3388	94.8	185	5.2
	>2500gr	36375	97.8	821	2.2
maternal education	no education	1907	96.7	66	3.3
	any primary	11764	96.7	398	3.3
	any secondary	21576	97.7	503	2.3
	higher secondary	6263	98.4	101	1.6
residence	rural	1251	98.9	14	1.1
	semi-urban	2236	99.0	23	1.0
	urban	18740	97.1	566	2.9
	metropolitan	11122	97.9	234	2.1

* Exludes children with missing DAZ or missing factor

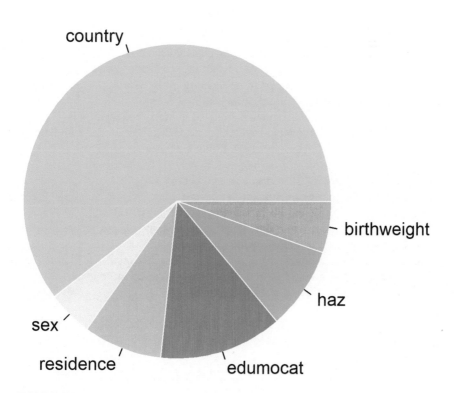

FIGURE 2.8.2   Relative importance of the explanatory factors in this study.

2.9 Discussion

Iris Eekhout[1]
Stef van Buuren[1,2]
[1]Netherlands Organisation for Applied Scientific Research TNO, Leiden, 2316 ZL, The Netherlands
[2]University of Utrecht, Utrecht, 3584 CH, The Netherlands

This closing section briefly summarizes the key lessons from previous sections. The section covers:

- D-score from multiple instruments (2.9.1)
- Variability within and between cohorts (2.9.2)
- D-score for international comparisons (2.9.3)
- Better measurement (2.9.4)

2.9.1 D-SCORE FROM MULTIPLE INSTRUMENTS

We developed the initial D-score methodology for just one instrument. In practice, however, we need to deal with data collected on multiple, partially overlapping tools. This chapter addressed the problem *how to define and calculate the D-score based on data coming from various sources, using multiple instruments administered at varying ages.*

We had longitudinal data available from 16 cohorts, collected with 15 tools to measure child development at various ages. Our analytic strategy to define a D-score from these data consists of the following steps:

1. Make an inventory of instruments and cohorts;
2. Combine all measurements into one dataset;
3. Find out which shared instruments connect cohorts;
4. Place similar items from different instruments into equate groups;
5. Find the best set of *active* equate groups;
6. Estimate item difficulty using a restricted Rasch model that requires the estimates of all items within an active equate group to be identical;
7. Weed out items that do not fit the model.

We need to perform steps 5, 6 and 7 in an iterative fashion. Depending on the result, we may also need to redefine, combine or break up equate groups (step 4).

These techniques are well-known within psychometrics and educational research. Our approach builds upon a well-grounded and robust theory of

DOI: 10.1201/9781003216315-20

170

psychological measurement. We, therefore, expect that repeating our method on other data will lead to very similar results.

A novel aspect in our methodology is the systematic formation of candidate equate groups by subject-matter experts based on similarity in concept and content. Our subsequent testing and tailoring of each equate group given the data provide empirical evidence of its quality for connecting instruments. While anchoring tests by itself is not novel, we are not aware of any work aimed at identifying the best set of active equate groups on this scale.

2.9.2   VARIABILITY WITHIN AND BETWEEN COHORTS

The final model retains 565 items and employs 18 equate groups. Given the difficulty estimates from that model, we can estimate the D-score and DAZ for each measurement.

Figure 2.6.1 reveals that all cohorts show a rapidly rising age trend in the D-score, which matches the earlier finding that child development is faster in younger children.

Figure 2.6.2 shows large overlaps in the DAZ distributions between cohorts. This finding suggests that the level of child development is similar in different regions of the world. Some studies display more variability in DAZ than others, which is likely to be related to differences in measurement error, as the number of milestones differs widely.

Observe that we used all cohorts for modelling, which may have made them appear more similar than they are. It would be good if we could verify the apparent similarities in level and variability of child development in different regions by other data that were not part of the modelling.

2.9.3   D-SCORE FOR INTERNATIONAL COMPARISONS

The D-score is a universal scale of early child development. The D-score does not depend on a particular instrument. Instead, we can calculate a D-score as long as appropriate difficulty estimates are available for the tool at hand. This feature makes the D-score methodology flexible and helpful for international comparisons.

Of course, the ideal situation for international comparisons would be that all countries collect child development data in the same way. In practice, this ideal may be difficult to achieve. Also, we cannot change past data. In these less-than-ideal worlds, the D-score presents a convenient, conscientious and timely alternative.

As an example, we outlined a generic strategy on how to advance on SDG 4.2.1. We use the D-score to operationalize the concept As an example, we outlined a generic strategy on how to advance on SDG 4.2.1. We use the D-score to operationalize the concept *developmentally on track*. We calculated age-conditional references of the D-score, analogous to the WHO Multicentre Growth Reference Study. We may then define cut-off values. Children above the cut-off then count as developmentally on track.

While we highlighted the principles, much work still needs to be done. First, there are over 150 instruments for child development, and our current key covers only a fraction of these. We are actively expanding the key using additional data, so as time passes the coverage of tools will go up. Second, we calculated the references on a mix of studies, some of which include special populations. Thus, we cannot interpret the current reference values as portraying normal development. We hope that the inclusion of healthy population data will improve the usefulness of the references as a standard for child development.

2.9.4   BETTER MEASUREMENT

The D-score metric is a generic measure of child development. It summarizes child development by *one number*. We found that D-score fairly represents development domains over the entire scale. Due to its generic nature, the D-score is less suitable for measuring a specific domain. It may then be better to use a specialized tool that accesses motor, cognitive or communication faculties. For example, think of sub-scales from the Bayley, ASQ, Griffiths, and so on. Note that also in those cases, one still has the option of calculating a D-score.

The opposite scenario may also be of interest. Suppose we want to measure generic development AND identify any areas of slow growth. Extending the measurement by adding more items from domains with a higher failure rate will then increase precision in areas of suspected delay.

Since we based the D-score on a statistical model, we may create instruments customized to the exact needs of the study. Population-based studies may require a short measure consisting of a handful of items per child, and aggregate scores over many children to achieve precision. Intervention studies aim for a precise estimate for the intervention effect. If group sizes are small, we may administer a more extended test to achieve the same precision and vice versa. At the other end of the spectrum, for clinical purposes, we want a precise estimate for one particular person, so here we will administer a relatively long test. The good news is: As long as we pick items from the statistical model, the D-score in those three cases are all values on the same scale.

Our ongoing work targets tailoring instruments to a study design and discusses all of these options. And more.

2.10 Appendices

Iris Eekhout[1]
Stef van Buuren[1,2]
[1]Netherlands Organisation for Applied
Scientific Research TNO, Leiden, 2316 ZL,
The Netherlands
[2]University of Utrecht, Utrecht, 3584 CH, The
Netherlands

A

Abbreviations

Section	Abbreviation	Description
2.2.2	GCDG-BGD-7MO	The Bangladesh study of the GCDG (Tofail *et al.*, 2008)
2.2.2	GCDG-BRA-1	The Brazil 1 study of the GCDG (Victora *et al.*, 2006)
2.2.2	GCDG-BRA-2	The Brazil 2 study of the GCDG (Moura *et al.*, 2010)
2.2.2	GCDG-CHL-1	The Chile 1 study of the GCDG (Lozoff *et al.*, 2003)
2.2.2	GCDG-CHL-2	The Chile 2 study of the GCDG (Conteras & González, 2015)
2.2.2	GCDG-CHN	The China study of the GCDG (Lozoff *et al.*, 2016)
2.2.2	GCDG-COL-LT45M	The Colombia 1 study of the GCDG (Attanasio *et al.*, 2014)
2.2.2	GCDG-COL-LT42M	The Colombia 2 study of the GCDG (Rubio-Codina *et al.*, 2016)
2.2.2	GCDG-ECU	The Ecuador study of the GCDG (Paxson & Schady, 2010)
2.2.2	GCDG-ETH	The Ethiopia study of the GCDG (Hanlon *et al.*, 2009)
2.2.2	GCDG-JAM-LBW	The Jamaica 1 study of the GCDG (Walker *et al.*, 2004)
2.2.2	GCDG-JAM-STUNTED	The Jamaica 2 study of the GCDG (Grantham-McGregor *et al.*, 1991)
2.2.2	GCDG-MDG	The Madagascar study of the GCDG (Fernald *et al.*, 2011)
2.2.2	GCDG-NLD-SMOCC	The Netherlands 1 study of the GCDG (Herngreen *et al.*, 1992)
2.2.2	GCDG-NLD-2	The Netherlands 2 study of the GCDG (Doove, 2010)
2.2.2	GCDG-ZAF	The South Africa study of the GCDG (Richter *et al.*, 2007)
2.2.3	by1	Bayley Scale for Infant and Todler Development version 1 (Bayley, 1969)
2.2.3	by2	Bayley Scale for Infant and Todler Development version 2 (Bayley, 1993)
2.2.3	by3	Bayley Scale for Infant and Todler Development version 3 (Bayley, 2006)
2.2.3	den	Denver Developmental Screening Test (Frankenburg *et al.*, 1992)
2.2.3	gri	Griffiths Mental Development Scales (Griffiths, 1967)
2.2.3	bat	Battelle Developmental Inventory (Newborg, 2005)
2.2.3	vin	Vineland Social Maturity Scale (Doll, 1953)

(Continued)

DOI: 10.1201/9781003216315-21

A

(Continued)

Section	Abbreviation	Description
2.2.3	ddi	Dutch Developmental Instrument (Schlesinger-Was, 1981)
2.2.3	bar	Barrera Moncada (Moncada, 1981)
2.2.3	tep	Test de Desarrollo Psicomotor (Haeussler & Marchant, 1999)
2.2.3	aqi	Ages and Stages Questionnaire (Squires & Bricker, 2009)
2.2.3	sbi	Stanford Binet Intelligence Scales (Roid, 2003)

B

Notation

Section	Symbol	Term	Description
2.4.4	β_n	Ability	True (but unknown) developmental score of child n
2.4.4	δ_I	Difficulty	True (but unknown) difficulty of item i
2.4.4	δ_q	Difficulty	The combined difficulty of the items in equate group q
2.4.4	π_{ni}	Probability	True (but unknown) probability that child n passes item i
2.4.4	l	Count	The number of items in the equate group
2.4.4	w_i	Count	The number of respondents with an observed score on item i
2.4.6	P_{ni}	Probability	Estimated probability that child n passes item i
2.4.6	x_{ni}	Data	Observed response of child n on item i, 0 or 1
2.4.6	W_{ni}	Variance	Variance of x_{ni}
2.4.6	z_{ni}	Residual	Standardized residual between x_{ni} and P_{ni}
2.4.6	N_i	Count	Number of responses on item i
2.5.6	r	Correlation	Correlation coefficient
2.6	D	Score	Developmental score of a child: D-score
2.6.2	sem	Error	Standard Error of Measurement: precision of the D-score

Data availability

UNDERLYING DATA

The raw data needed to replicate these analyses are not public, so we cannot share it with this publication. However, the reader can apply for access to the data through the study contact. The table given below contains the contact information for each cohort included in this publication.

A subset of studies made their study data publicly available under a CC BY 4.0 license (https://creativecommons.org/licenses/by/4.0/)[1]. Authorship remains with the study coordinator, but users are free to redistribute, alter and combine the data, on the condition of giving appropriate credit with any redistributions of the material. The URL of the public data is https://d-score.org/childdevdata/.

Name in publication	Reference	Contact
GCDG-BGD-7MO	Hamadani *et al.*, 2011; Tofail, 2009	Jena Hamadani (jena@icddrb.org)
GCDG-BRA-1	Halpern *et al.*, 1996; Victora *et al.*, 2006	Simone Karam (Karam.simone@gmail.com)
GCDG-BRA-2	Moura *et al.*, 2010	Simone Karam (Karam.simone@gmail.com)
GCDG-CHL-1	Lozoff *et al.*, 2013	Betsy Lozoff (blozoff@umich.edu)
GCDG-CHL-2	Conteral & González, 2015	Lia Fernald (fernald@berkeley.edu)
GCDG-CHN	Angulo-Barroso *et al.*, 2016; Lozoff *et al.*, 2016; Santos *et al.*, 2017	Betsy Lozoff (blozoff@umich.edu)
GCDG-COL-LT45M	Andrew *et al.*, 2017; Attanasio *et al.*, 2014	Marta Rubio (martarubio@iadb.org)
GCDG-COL-LT42M	Rubio-Codina *et al.*, 2016	Marta Rubio (martarubio@iadb.org)
GCDG-ECU	Araujo *et al.*, 2016; Fernald & Hidrobo, 2011; Paxon & Shady, 2010	Caridad Araujo (mcaraujo@iadb.org)
GCDG-ETH	Hanlon *et al.*, 2016	Charlotte Hanlon (charlotte.hanlon@kcl.ac.uk)
GCDG-JAM-LBW	Walker *et al.*, 2004; Walker *et al.*, 2010	Susan Walker (susan.walker@uwimona.edu.jm)

(Continued)

Name in publication	Reference	Contact
GCDG-JAM-STUNTED	Grantham-McGregor *et al.*, 1991; Grantham-McGregor *et al.*, 1997; Walker *et al.*, 2005	Susan Walker (susan.walker@uwimona.edu.jm)
GCDG-MDG	Galasso *et al.*, 2011; Galasso *et al.*, 2017	Ann Weber (annweber@stanford.edu)
GCDG-NLD-SMOCC	Herngreen *et al.*, 1992	Paul Verkerk (paul.verkerk@tno.nl)
GCDG-NLD-2	Doove *et al.*, 2010; Doove *et al.*, 2019;	Bernice Doove (bernice.doove@maastrichtuniversity.nl)
GCDG-ZAF	Richter *et al.*, 1995; Richter *et al.*, 2004; Richter *et al.*, 2007; Yach *et al.*, 1991	Linda Richter (Linda.Richter@wits.ac.za)

Acknowledgements

This chapter was supported by the Bill & Melinda Gates Foundation. The contents are the sole responsibility of the authors and may not necessarily represent the official views of the Bill & Melinda Gates Foundation or other agencies that may have supported the primary data studies used in the present chapter. The authors wish to recognize the principal investigators and their study team members for their generous contribution of the data that were used to illustrate this booklet and the members of the Global Child Development Group who directly or indirectly contributed to the contents of this chapter: Maureen M. Black, Gary L. Darmstadt, M. Caridad Araujo, Susan M. Changm, Bernice M. Doove, Lia C.H. Fernald, Emanuela Galasso, Sally Grantham-McGregor, Pamela Jervis, Jena D. Hamadani, Charlotte Hanlon, Simone M. Karam, Betsy Lozoff, Orazio Attanasio, Girmay Medhin, Ana M. B. Menezes and the 1993 Pelotas cohort team, Helen Pitchik, Lisy Ratsifandrihamanana, Sarah Reynolds, Linda Richter, Marta Rubio-Codina, Norbert Schady, Susan P. Walker, Ann M. Weber.

Note

[1] Zenodo: D-score/childdevdata: childdevdata 1.0.1, http://doi.org/10.5281/zenodo.4685979 (van Buuren, 2021)

References

Attanasio OP, Fernández C, Fitzsimons EOA, *et al.*: Using the infrastructure of a conditional cash transfer program to deliver a scalable integrated early child development program in Colombia: cluster randomized controlled trial. *BMJ.* 2014; 349: g5785. 2526622210.1136/bmj.g57854179481

Bayley N: Bayley Scales of Infant Development. 1969. Reference Source

Bayley N: The Bayley Scales of Infant Development-II. 1993. Reference Source

Bayley N: Bayley Scales of Infant and Toddler Development–Third Edition: Technical Manual. 2006. Reference Source

Bellman M, Byrne O, Sege R: Developmental Assessment of Children. *BMJ.* 2013; 346 (e8687): e8687. 10.1136/bmj.e8687

Borghi E, de Onis M, Garza C, *et al.*: Construction of the World Health Organization child growth standards: selection of methods for attained growth curves. *Stat Med.* 2006; 25(2): 247–265. 1614396810.1002/sim.2227

Britto PR, Lye SJ, Proulx K, *et al.*: Nurturing Care: Promoting Early Childhood Development. *Lancet.* 2017; 389(10064): 91–102. 2771761510.1016/S0140-6736 (16)31390-3

Conteras D, González S: Determinants of early child development in Chile: Health, cognitive and demographic factors. *Int J Educ Dev.* 2015; 40: 217–230. 10.1016/j. ijedudev.2014.06.010

Doll EA: The Measurement of Social Competence: A Manual for the Vineland Social Maturity Scale. 1953. 10.1037/11349-000

Doove BM: Ontwikkeling kinderen in Maastricht en Heuvelland (MOM), Evaluatie integraal kindvolgsysteem voor signalering in de Jeugdgezondheidszorg: MOMknowsbest. 2010. Reference Source

Fernald LCH, Prado E, Kariger P, *et al.*: A Toolkit for Measuring Early Childhood Development in Low and Middle-Income Countries. 2017. Reference Source

Fernald LCH, Weber A, Galasso E, *et al.*: Socioeconomic gradients and child development in a very low income population: evidence from Madagascar. *Dev Sci.* 2011; 14(4): 832–847. 2167610210.1111/j.1467-7687.2010.01032.x

Frankenburg WK, Dodds J, Archer P, *et al.*: The Denver II: A Major Revision and Restandardization of the Denver Developmental Screening Test. *Pediatrics.* 1992; 89(1): 91–97. 137018510.1542/peds.89.1.91

Frankenburg WK, Dodds J, Archer P, *et al.*: The DENVER II Technical Manual. 1990.

Gesell A: *Infant and Child in the Culture of Today* . Los Angeles, CA: Read Book Ltd, 1943. Reference Source

Grantham-McGregor SM, Powell CA, Walker SP, *et al.*: Nutritional supplementation, psychosocial stimulation, and mental development of stunted children: the Jamaican Study. *Lancet.* 1991; 338(8758): 1–5. 167608310.1016/0140-6736(91)90001-6

Griffiths R: The Abilities of Babies: A Study in Mental Measurement. 1967. Reference Source

Haeussler IM, Marchant T: Tepsi: Test de Desarrollo Psicomotor 2-5 años. 1999.

Hagen E, Stattler J: Stanford–Binet Intelligence Scales, Fourth Edition. 1986.

Hanlon C, Medhin G, Alem A, *et al.*: Impact of antenatal common mental disorders upon perinatal outcomes in Ethiopia: the P-MaMiE population-based cohort study.

Trop Med Int Health. 2009; 14(2): 156–166. 1918751410.1111/j.1365-3156.2008.02198.x

Herngreen WP, Reerink JD, van Noord-Zaadstra BM, *et al.*: SMOCC: Design of a Representative Cohort-study of Live-born Infants in the Netherlands. *Eur J Public Health.* 1992; 2(2): 117–122. 10.1093/eurpub/2.2.117

Jacobusse G, van Buuren S, Verkerk PH: An Interval Scale for Development of Children Aged 0-2 Years. *Stat Med.* 2006; 25(13): 2272–2283. 1614399510.1002/sim.2351

Kim SH, Cohen AS: A Comparison of Linking and Concurrent Calibration Under Item Response Theory. *Appl Psychol Meas.* 1998; 22(2): 131–143. 10.1177/01466216980222003

Loizillon A, Petrowski N, Britto P, *et al.*: Development of the Early Childhood Development Index in MICS Surveys. MICS Methodological Papers, No. 6. Data and Analytics Section, Division of Data. *Research and Policy.* New York: UNICEF, 2017. Reference Source

Lozoff B, De Andraca I, Castillo M, *et al.*: Behavioral and developmental effects of preventing iron-deficiency anemia in healthy full-term infants. *Pediatrics.* 2003; 112(4): 846–854. 14523176

Lozoff B, Jiang Y, Li X, *et al.*: Low-Dose Iron Supplementation in Infancy Modestly Increases Infant Iron Status at 9 Mo without Decreasing Growth or Increasing Illness in a Randomized Clinical Trial in Rural China. *J Nutr.* 2016; 146(3): 612–621. 2679155610.3945/jn.115.2239174763485

Moncada GB: Crecimiento y Desarrollo Psicológico Del Niño Venezolano. 1981. Reference Source

Moura DR, Costa JC, Santos IS, *et al.*: Natural history of suspected developmental delay between 12 and 24 months of age in the 2004 Pelotas birth cohort. *J Paediatr Child Health.* 2010; 46(6): 329–336. 2041241010.1111/j.1440-1754.2010.01717.x

Newborg J: Battelle Developmental Inventory-2nd Edition. 2005.

Paxson C, Schady N: Does money matter? The effects of cash transfers on child development in rural Ecuador. *Econ Dev Cult Change.* 2010; 59(1): 187–229. 2082189610.1086/655458

Richter L, Norris S, Pettifor J, *et al.*: Cohort Profile: Mandela's children: the 1990 Birth to Twenty study in South Africa. *Int J Epidemiol.* 2007; 36(3): 504–511. 1735597910.1093/ije/dym0162702039

Roid GH: Stanford–Binet Intelligence Scales, Fifth Edition. 2003. Reference Source

Rubio-Codina M, Araujo MC, Attanasio O, *et al.*: Concurrent Validity and Feasibility of Short Tests Currently Used to Measure Early Childhood Development in Large Scale Studies. Edited by David O.Carpenter.*PLoS One.* 2016; 11(8): e0160962. 2754863410.1371/journal.pone.01609624993374

Schlesinger-Was EA: Ontwikkelingsonderzoek van Zuigelingen En Kleuters Op Het Consultatiebureau. 1981. Reference Source

Shirley MM: *The First Two Years: A Study of Twenty-Five Babies. Vol. II: Intellectual Development* . Minneapolis: University of Minnesota Press, 1933. Reference Source

Squires J, Bricker D: Ages & Stages Questionnaires, Third Edition (ASQ-3) . A Parent-Completed Child-Monitoring System. 2009. Reference Source

Tofail F, Persson LA, El Arifeen S, *et al.*: Effects of prenatal food and micronutrient supplementation on infant development: a randomized trial from the Maternal and Infant Nutrition Interventions, Matlab (MINIMat) study. *Am J Clin Nutr.* 2008; 87 (3): 704–711. 1832661010.1093/ajcn/87.3.704

van Buuren S: Growth Charts of Human Development. *Stat Methods Med Res*. 2014; 23 (4): 346–368. 2348701910.1177/0962280212473300

van Buuren S: D-score/childdevdata: childdevdata 1.0.1. (Version v1.0.1). *Zenodo*. 2021. http://www.doi.org/10.5281/zenodo.4685979

van Buuren S, Eekhout I: Child development with the D-score: turning milestones into measurement. *F1000Res*. (in press). 2021. Reference Source

Verloove-Vanhorick SP, Verwey RA, Brand R, *et al.*: Neonatal mortality risk in relation to gestational age and birthweight. Results of a national survey of preterm and very-low-birthweight infants in the Netherlands. *Lancet*. 1986; 1(8472): 55–57. 286731210.1016/s0140-6736(86)90713-0

Victora CG, Araújo CLP, Menezes AMB, *et al.*: Methodological aspects of the 1993 Pelotas (Brazil) Birth Cohort Study. *Rev Saude Publica*. 2006; 40(1): 39–46. 1641098110.1590/s0034-89102006000100008291767

Walker SP, Chang SM, Powell CA, *et al.*: Psychosocial intervention improves the development of term low-birth-weight infants. *J Nutr*. 2004; 134(6): 1417–1423. 1517340610.1093/jn/134.6.1417

Weber AM, Rubio-Codina M, Walker SP, *et al.*: The D-score: A Metric for Interpreting the Early Development of Infants and Toddlers Across Global Settings. *BMJ Glob Health*. 2019; 4(6): e001724. 3180350810.1136/bmjgh-2019-0017246882553

Wright BD, Masters GN: *Rating Scale Analysis: Rasch Measurement*. Chicago: MESA Press, 1982. Reference Source

Index